MANAGING DIABETICS PROPERLY

MANAGING DIABETICS PROPERLY

NURSING79 BOOKS
Intermed Communications, Inc.
Horsham, Pa.

NURSING79 BOOKS

PUBLISHER: Eugene W. Jackson
Editorial Director: Daniel L. Cheney
Clinical Director: Margaret Van Meter, RN
Circulation Director: Ronald S. Moyer

NURSING SKILLBOOK™ SERIES
SERIES EDITOR: Patricia S. Chaney
Researcher: Avery Rome
Copy Editor: Patricia A. Hamilton
Production Manager: Bernard Haas
Production Assistants: Dave Kosten, Margie Tyson
Designer: Sally Collins
Art Assistants: Maggie Arnott, Patricia Wertz,
　　　　　　　　　Owen G. Heinrich

Cover and divider illustrations by John Freas
Text illustrations by Jack Crane

Text and information on dead space (pp. 54-55) adapted from
Diabetes Forecast, courtesy of Patricia A. Lawrence, RN, MA,
and Margaret Gebhardt, RPh, and the American Diabetes
Association.

Library of Congress cataloging in publication data.

Main entry under title:

MANAGING DIABETICS PROPERLY

"Nursing Skillbook series."
Includes index.
1. Diabetes.　　2. Diabetes — Nursing.
RC660.M34 1977b　　610.73'6　　78-25770
ISBN 0-916730-0-4-2

CONTENTS

FOREWORD

DIABETES IS an old disease — with a new interest and new involvement for nurses. When insulin was discovered in 1920, the medical world assumed that it was "taken care of." So it was all but forgotten — forgotten, that is, until diabetics of long-standing started developing complications and problems. It became a major medical problem again — a chronic problem that still affects more than 10 million people in the U.S. alone.

No matter what your field, you can't forget diabetes. Whether you work in a newborn nursery, a hospital, a nursing home, or a community agency, you'll see diabetics in your practice. Even if the diabetes itself isn't your main focus in nursing, it's bound to affect your care of a diabetic's other medical problems.

But your involvement with diabetes runs deeper than with most diseases. For years nurses have used diabetes as their model when caring for someone with a chronic disease. Then, when nurses began acting as primary care givers, diabetes was one of the first chronic diseases for which they developed protocols. Today, as the emphasis of health care shifts from episodic care to prevention, nurses are becoming even more deeply involved as patient educators. In short, nurses are getting a chance to act independently in the care of diabetics.

They're delivering primary care and teaching patients to live with and manage their disease within their own lifestyles.

For all of these reasons, you may want to sharpen your skills in caring for diabetics. *Managing Diabetics Properly* addresses itself to the basic knowledge you'll need to care for patients with diabetes, whether diabetes is their major medical problem or just an adjunct to their major medical problem. This book starts with recognition — an important first step since you are apt to be the first member of the health team to recognize the symptoms of diabetes. It thoroughly covers treatment, not only for the average diabetic but also for those with special problems such as blindness, pregnancy, or surgery — another vital step since you have to work with the doctor to plan an appropriate daily routine for each new diabetic. And it covers patient education — perhaps your greatest role in diabetes.

Managing Diabetics Properly presents the most up-to-date material on diabetes. And it builds on itself. At the end of each section, you'll find a "Skillcheck" that helps you synthesize all the material you've just read, and apply it to your particular practice.

Diabetes doesn't have to be a problem for you; instead, it should be a nursing challenge. By developing an understanding of diabetics' emotional and physical needs, you can better care for them in both chronic and acute settings. It's a challenging, rewarding way to deliver nursing care.

—BARBARA CHRISTMAN, RN, MSN
President, American Association of
Diabetes Educators
Member, Board of Trustees,
American Diabetes Association

HOW TO RECOGNIZE AND TREAT DIABETES

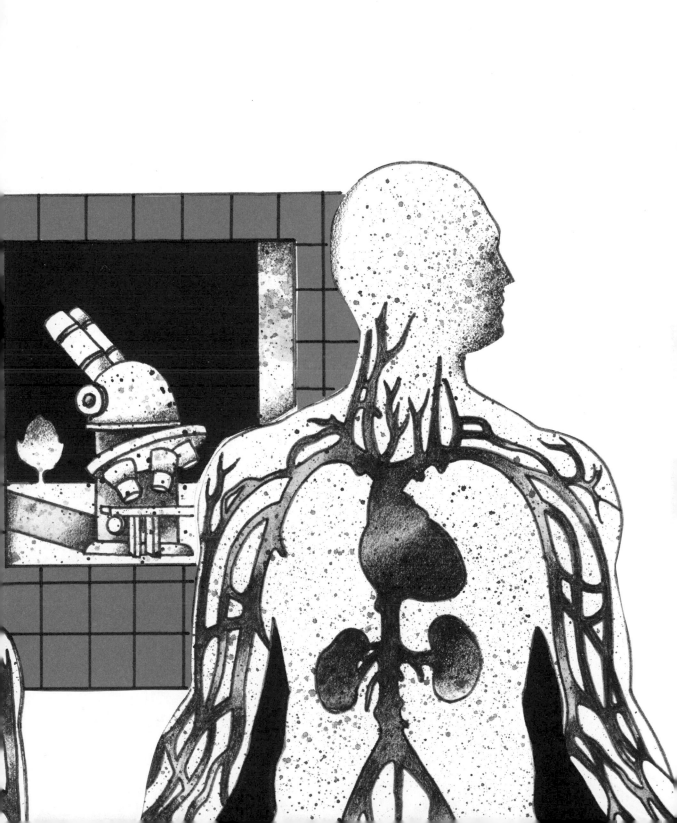

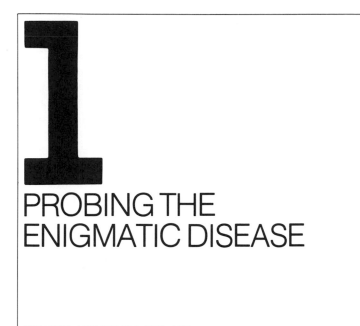

1
PROBING THE ENIGMATIC DISEASE

BY RITA NEMCHIK, RN, MS

JUST WHAT is diabetes? Think about it for a minute; actually take time to answer the question.

Now, examine your answer. Did you find yourself describing it in terms of metabolism? In terms of insufficient insulin and elevated blood glucose levels? If you're a typical nurse, you probably did. And technically your answer may be perfectly correct. But I wonder if it was extensive enough...if it was *practical*. Think again: Would your answer help a diabetic manage his disease better?

Unfortunately it's probably only a start. Because we nurses and most practitioners are accustomed to viewing diabetes clinically. Yet to a diabetic, particularly a new insulin-dependent diabetic, the disease is something much more fundamental — an ongoing threat to his financial status, to his life-style, and to his very life. And to give him practical help in managing his diabetes, you must approach it from *his* perspective.

That's not always easy, even if you often work with diabetics or are a diabetic yourself, as I am. I remember one of my patients who had just learned of his diabetes and seemed very upset. Based on my experience, I immediately assumed that he was concerned about some part of his therapy. So, I reviewed his diet and insulin injections over and over again. He

The pancreas — the secret of it all
The pancreas is a three- to four-inch gland shaped like a triangle. The islets of Langerhans, which produce the body's insulin, drain directly into the bloodstream and help maintain glucose levels in the blood.

still seemed upset. Only later did I discover why: His real concern wasn't diet and insulin therapy but rather impotence, which had been his first symptom of diabetes. Fortunately his wife finally explained his concern to me so the doctor and I could help him deal with it. If his wife hadn't intervened, though, I'm sure that man would have taken a long time to adjust to his condition — thanks to the interference of my own perspective.

That story underlines what I believe is the most important precept of nursing for diabetic patients: To help a new diabetic cope with his diagnosis, you have to develop not only a clinical appreciation of diabetes but also a practical perspective. The balance of this book is devoted to the practical side of diabetes. When you finish reading it, you should be better able to truly help your patients manage their diabetes.

But with diabetes, as with all diseases, practice must be grounded in clinical theory. So let's get back to my original question: Just what is diabetes? To help you understand it practically, here's a brief clinical explanation.

The enigmatic disease
Simply stated, diabetes is a chronic systemic disease whose chief manifestations include disorders in the metabolism of insulin, carbohydrates, fats, and proteins and in the structure and function of blood vessels. Early signs and symptoms of the disease stem from the metabolic disorders; later complications stem from the vascular disorders.

Although the etiology of diabetes still baffles investigators, the primary pathology lies in a deficiency in insulin secretion. Metabolically, insulin is responsible for increasing the storage of energy-yielding fuels in the liver, muscle, and adipose tissues. The body relies on carbohydrates as its chief fuel; when we eat carbohydrates, insulin converts them to the fuel known as glucose, some of which is stored until it is needed. Lacking enough insulin, though, the body will begin to rely on fats as its chief fuel. As by-products of this metabolism, fats produce ketones (acetone, acetoacetic acid, and betahydroxybutyric acid) which lead to diabetic acidosis.

In nondiabetic persons, the blood-sugar itself regulates the rate of insulin secretion. Normally, carbohydrates increase the blood-sugar level, stimulating the beta cells in the islets of the pancreas to release insulin in two stages: an initial rapid

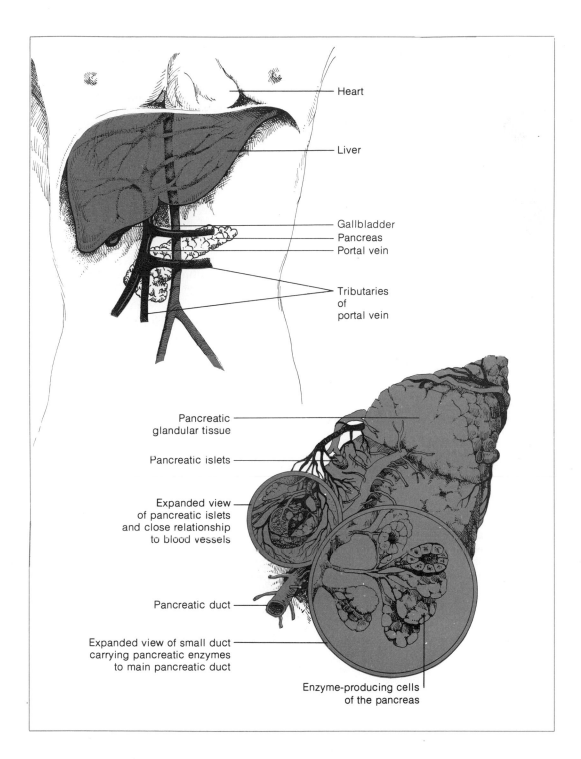

Heart

Liver

Gallbladder
Pancreas
Portal vein

Tributaries
of
portal vein

Pancreatic
glandular tissue

Pancreatic islets

Expanded view
of pancreatic islets
and close relationship
to blood vessels

Pancreatic duct

Expanded view of small duct
carrying pancreatic enzymes
to main pancreatic duct

Enzyme-producing cells
of the pancreas

output, followed by a second gradual output. As the blood-sugar level falls, the beta cell stimulus diminishes. When the blood-sugar level falls below normal, the alpha cells in the pancreas secrete glucagon, a hyperglycemic agent that fosters the conversion of liver starch (glycogen) to glucose and thus raises the blood-sugar level. Thus, the body maintains its stasis. In diabetes, this process goes awry.

In mild cases of diabetes, the deficiency of insulin leads to inadequate utilization of ingested carbohydrates and disposal of converted glucose. In more severe cases, it also leads to overproduction of glucose, loss of body fat, and dissipation of protein reserves. Besides the insulin deficiency, diabetes may cause an abnormally high secretion of glucagon, which raises the blood-sugar level even higher. The consequent hyperglycemia can spiral upward from the normal blood glucose levels of 80 to 120 mg/100 ml to more than 1000 mg/100 ml. The powerful osmotic force of the elevated blood sugar draws cellular water into the blood, depleting both water and the body's sugar stores through the kidneys: Electrolytes, particularly potassium, are lost too.

Seeing before feeling

The above mechanism produces the surest signs of diabetes: Hyperglycemia, polyuria, polydipsia, polyphagia, and weight loss. Long before these conclusive signs appear, though, other warning signs may arise.

Common early warning signals involve the skin, in the form of shin spots, recurrent infections, or recalcitrant fungal infections.

Shin spots, which occur more often in men than in women, may develop from a blow on the shin. A brown, distinct spot about the size of a penny appears on the front of the shin.

Recurrent infections include boils, carbuncles, and furuncles. Although these appear most often on the posterior neck, they can develop anywhere on the body.

Recalcitrant fungal infections develop between toes or in nail beds. True, nondiabetics may develop the same infections. But people prone to diabetes seem particularly susceptible to them.

Pregnancy also can trigger some early warning signs in a diabetes-prone woman. She may develop complications, such as toxemia or premature deliveries, which commonly occur among diabetics. Or, she may deliver a heavy baby, often more than 10 pounds. Or, she may actually develop hyperglycemia for the duration of her pregnancy (gestational diabetes). Although her blood sugar might return to normal after delivery, she might have to control it with insulin during pregnancy just as a diabetic of long standing.

Obesity also can be a sign of impending diabetes. Since obesity decreases tissue responsiveness to insulin and thus increases the demand for insulin, it contributes to abnormal insulin secretion in a person who is genetically predisposed to diabetes.

Strangely enough, hypoglycemia, which is the direct opposite of diabetes, also can be a sign of impending hyperglycemia or early diabetes in an adult. Usually the symptoms of hypoglycemia (tremors, sweating, headache, fatigue, and faintness) appear 3 to 5 hours after the person has eaten. What happens is this: After eating a glucose load, the patient has a sluggish insulin response. So, for the first couple of hours after eating, his blood glucose level is quite high. In response to the excessive glucose, his pancreas finally sends forth an excessive dose of insulin, which eventually lowers the glucose level well below normal.

Finally, many of the complications of diabetes (see Chapter 10) may develop before the diabetes itself is apparent. These early warnings include eye changes, kidney dysfunction, numbness and tingling in the feet or legs, vascular disease, and hardening of the arteries.

If any of these early warning signs appear, particularly any combination of them, you might be wise to advise a patient to have a blood-sugar test. Sometimes a glucose tolerance test is needed to confirm the diagnosis.

Kids are different

Of course, most of the early signs occur only in adult-onset or maturity-onset diabetics — those who develop the disease later in life (usually after the age of 30, although sometimes earlier). This milder form of diabetes, which comes on gradually, is by far the most common, accounting for 90% of the diabetic population. All adult-onset diabetics usually can produce some insulin. In fact, some may have normal or even elevated insulin production, but their bodies just can't use the insulin efficiently. With insufficient insulin or inefficient use of

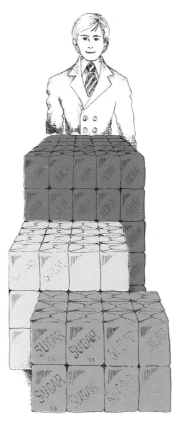

Annual sugar loss in diabetics
An untreated severe diabetic loses the equivalent of 109 five-pound bags of sugar in his urine every year, represented by the dark brown stack of bags in the background. An untreated moderate diabetic loses the equivalent of 48 five-pound sugar bags, as indicated by the light brown stack in the middle ground, and an untreated mild diabetic loses the equivalent of 28 five-pound sugar bags, as shown by the medium brown stack in the foreground.

TABLE 1 — DIFFERENCE BETWEEN JUVENILE-ONSET AND ADULT-ONSET DIABETES

	Juvenile Type	Adult Type
Age of onset	Frequently before 20 years but can be after 20	Usually after 30 but sometimes before 30
Type of onset	Abrupt	Gradual
Symptoms	Thirst, urinary frequency, increased appetite, weight loss	Sometimes none
Stability	Wide fluctuations of blood sugar with marked sensitivity to diet, exercise, and insulin	Usually easily controlled if patient adheres to a proper diet
Ketoacidosis	Frequent only if therapy is inadequate	Uncommon except with severe stress, infection, etc.
Hypoglycemia	More frequent	Uncommon
Control of diabetes	Difficult	Less difficult
Endogenous insulin	Absent	Present
Complications	May occur	May occur
Diet	Most important	Most important
Insulin	Needed by all	Needed by only 20 to 30%
Oral hypoglycemic agent	Not indicated	Useful for about 40%

it, the body can't convert ingested foods for energy or energy reserves. That's why adult-onset diabetics often feel exhausted and lose a great amount of weight before they discover their disease.

In a mild adult-onset diabetic, only a glucose tolerance test can detect the disease; a fasting blood-sugar test won't. The reason is that only the first, rapid phase of insulin output is impaired; the second, gradual phase remains normal. So, when the patient eats a glucose load, his body doesn't respond with a quick spurt of insulin. The glucose reaches the liver and peripheral tissues very slowly. After the initial onslaught of glucose, though, the body can produce enough insulin to accommodate the residual glucose.

Juvenile-onset diabetes presents quite a different picture. Although it can occur at any age, juvenile-onset diabetes usually develops during childhood or puberty. Because its hallmark is a total lack of insulin, it comes with stunning swiftness. Without any insulin, the child may go into ketoacidotic coma — sometimes the first clue to the child's

Stage	General characteristics	Glucose tolerance test	Fasting blood-sugar	Symptoms	Angiopathies
I. Prediabetes	No abnormal metabolism of glucose; can be diagnosed only in retrospect (after patient develops overt diabetes)	Normal	Normal	None	Rare
II. Subclinical (chemical)	Elevated blood-sugar levels only under stress (pregnancy; infections; injury; excess of adrenal, thyroid, or pituitary hormones, etc.)	Abnormal only during stress	Normal	None	Rare
III. Latent (chemical)	Abnormally elevated blood-sugar levels but no symptoms	Abnormal	Normal or abnormal	Uncommon	Possible
IV. Overt or frank	Abnormally elevated blood-sugar levels with symptoms	Abnormal	Abnormal	Common	Common

TABLE 2 — STAGES OF DIABETES AND THEIR CHARACTERISTICS

disease. Because juvenile diabetics must rely totally on exogenous insulin, they must get prompt treatment to control their labile condition. And because their condition is more serious and erratic than an adult-onset diabetic's, they're more prone to ketoacidosis, hypoglycemia, and hyperglycemic hyperosmolar nonketotic coma (HHNK).

Table 1 shows the basic differences between adult-onset and juvenile-onset diabetes.

Just a stage?

In addition to classifying diabetes by onset, you can classify it by degree or stage of abnormality. The stages are, in order of severity, pre diabetes, sub clinical diabetes, latent diabetes, and overt diabetes. A patient may progress through all stages, remain in one, or even revert to a less severe one. Table 2 outlines the basic distinctions between these stages. Of course, these stages are arbitrary. But they can help you alert a patient to possible difficulties.

Like the stages, the clinical definition of diabetes and the distinctions between juvenile-onset and adult-onset diabetes are merely convenient tools to help you understand this disease. Once a patient's diagnosis has been confirmed, the great

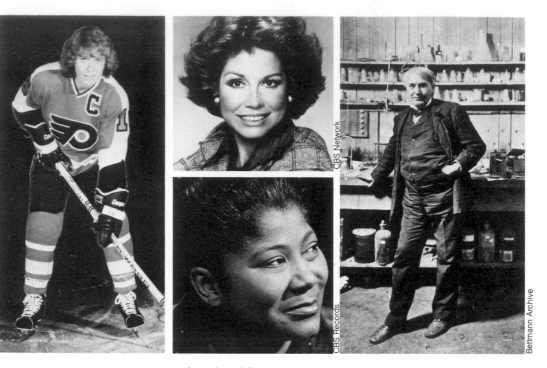

Philadelphia Flyers

CBS Network

CBS Records

Bettmann Archive

Famous diabetics
In educating a recently diagnosed diabetic, you can help alleviate his apprehensions by reminding him that today and throughout history many diabetics have reached fame, even in demanding vigorous careers. A few are Bobby Clarke, Mary Tyler Moore, Mahalia Jackson, Thomas Edison. Other diabetics include Jack Benny, Paul Cezanne, Nikita Krushchev, Mario Puzo, Jackie Robinson, Dan Rowan, Spencer Tracy, and H. G. Wells.

task at hand is to teach him to manage and to cope with it.

One last thing: Perhaps what diabetic patients need most is your encouragement and optimism. Years ago, the word diabetes evoked horror in many people because they knew someone who'd had severe complications of diabetes. Today, people seem a little more enlightened. Television spots showing famous personalities who have diabetes have done much to educate the public.

Still, a patient may be open-minded about the disease until he hears he has it. Then, his old fears may crop up again.

Throughout your teaching, emphasize that, with judicious self-care, he can live a nearly normal life. That bit of optimism, combined with your realistic instructions, will help him learn to handle his condition with practicality and wisdom.

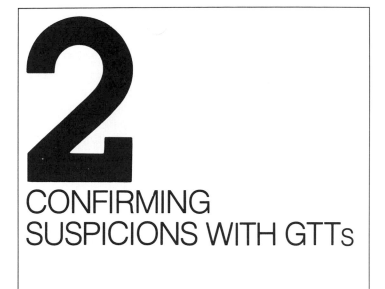

2

CONFIRMING SUSPICIONS WITH GTTs

BY MICHAEL L. O'CONNOR, MD

ALTHOUGH DIABETES SCREENING and diagnostic tests are simple procedures that give accurate results when done correctly, they can be misleading if the patient isn't properly prepared. That's where you come in. Since you're in the best position to monitor the patient's preparation, you can play an important role in determining the tests' reliability.

Screening tests for diabetes measure glucose in either urine or blood. Of these, the urine glucose measurement is the most simple, requiring no advance preparation. A Clinitest tablet is simply dropped into the patient's urine specimen and the resulting color indicates the concentration of glucose. But this test has limited value. In order for glucose to spill over into urine, the blood glucose concentration must exceed 130 to 140 mg/dl — well above the normal level.

The fasting blood glucose screening test has limited value because some patients with mild diabetes or adult-onset diabetes will pass this test with normal values. If the doctor orders it, though, be sure to advise the patient not to take food or any medications for eight hours before the test (an overnight fast).

Whenever possible, a 1- or 2-hour postprandial glucose measurement, which is done with a single blood sample, is the screening test of choice. After an overnight fast, the patient

Diseases that affect glucose tolerance
Patients recovering from severe illnesses or surgery should have glucose tolerance tests postponed. Here are some of the effects of some diseases.
Peripheral resistance to insulin: caused by diseases requiring prolonged bedrest, such as chronic neuromuscular disorders and hip fractures
Sluggish insulin response: caused by acute starvation states or malnutrition
Glucose intolerance: caused by acromegaly, Cushing's syndrome, potassium loss
Carbohydrate intolerance: caused by pheochromocytoma, hyperthyroidism

eats a meal of about 100 grams of carbohydrate (the glucose load). Then, 1 or 2 hours later, the blood sample is drawn.

In some hospitals, nurses draw the samples and send them to the laboratory for analysis, while in others the patient is sent to the laboratory for the procedure. Whichever is the policy in your hospital, you are responsible for seeing that the patient fasts and eats adequately at the appropriate times.

If the fasting blood sugar test shows a glucose level above 140 mg/dl or the postprandial test shows a glucose level above 200 mg/dl, the patient probably has diabetes; a diagnostic glucose tolerance test wouldn't tell you much more. But if the results of the screening test are "ambiguous" or "probable diabetes" (see Table), the patient should have a diagnostic oral glucose tolerance test. Also, certain types of patients who have higher incidences of diabetes than the general population are often given the diagnostic test rather than the screening test. These patients include:

• Those with a family history of diabetes
• Obese patients
• Those with transitory glycosuria or nondiagnostic hyperglycemia, especially during the course of pregnancy, surgical procedures, trauma, emotional stress, myocardial infarction, cerebrovascular accident, or administration of adrenal steroids
• Those with unexplained episodes of hypoglycemia
• Women who have delivered large babies or have had pregnancies resulting in abortions, premature labor, stillbirths, or neonatal deaths
• Those with unexplained neuropathy, retinopathy, nephropathy, or peripheral vascular disease
• Those who've had recurrent infections, especially boils, abscesses, and the like.

Generally, the diagnostic oral glucose tolerance test should be performed only on ambulatory patients who are not acutely ill or recovering from major surgery or acute illness. If an ill person is overtly diabetic, the 2-hour postprandial screening test will detect the diabetes. If it doesn't, the diagnostic test should be delayed until his metabolism has returned to normal — usually when he is ambulatory.

Patient preparation for this test is most important. Improper preparation is probably the greatest source of error in diabetes testing.

SERUM GLUCOSE mg/dl		
1-hr. PP	**2-hr. PP**	**Diagnosis**
Less than 150	Less than 120	Normal
150 to 185	120 to 140	Ambiguous
Greater than 185	Greater than 160	Probable diabetes
Greater than 200	Greater than 160	Clearly diabetes

Diet. Be sure the patient is on a normal diet with an intake of at least 300 grams of carbohydrates per day for 3 days preceding the test. When you describe the test procedure to the patient, stress the importance of his eating the loading diet. You can suggest that the patient eat his normal diet *plus* high-carbohydrate snacks at midmorning, midafternoon, and bedtime. Make the following exceptions, though: If the patient is grossly overweight and following a 300-Gm/day carbohydrate reducing diet, don't put him on the three-day preparatory diet. If the patient has been anorexic or eating poorly, put him on a preparatory diet for *seven* days.

Medication. See that all drugs proven or believed to influence the glucose tolerance test (e.g., hormones, salicylates, diuretic agents, and hypoglycemic agents) are discontinued for at least 3 days before the test. If a patient is on oral contraceptives, have her omit them for one cycle, if possible.

Fasting period. See that the patient has no food for at least 8 but not more than 16 hours preceding the test. He may have water, however.

Miscellaneous restrictions. Be sure that the patient avoids drinking coffee, smoking, and doing any unusual physical exercise for at least 8 hours before and during the test.

Again, depending on your hospital's policy, you may collect the specimens yourself or send the patient to the laboratory for the test. If the patient is to have the test done in the laboratory, you should see that he is dressed warmly and that he has something to occupy his time during the test (e.g., reading material, puzzles or games, handiwork, or the like).

The test should be conducted between 7 a.m. and 12 noon, with the fasting specimens (blood and urine) taken between 7 and 9 a.m. If the patient should be weighed before the test, be sure you actually weigh him — don't just ask him his weight.

If you're doing the test yourself, administer the oral glucose (loading dose) over several minutes in a dosage appropriate to the patient's age and body size ("ideal" weight is used for

Drugs that affect glucose tolerance
Some medications elevate blood glucose; others depress it. Here are some effects to keep in mind when you're assessing a patient's test results.
Elevate glucose:
diazoxide (Hyperstat), nicotinic acid (Nicalex), oral contraceptives containing mestranol (Enovid, Norinyl, Norquen, Ortho-Novum, Ortho-Novum SQ, Ovulen), phenytoin (Dilantin), systemic glucocorticoids, and thiazides and other potassium-depleting diuretics
Depress glucose:
alcohol, salicylates (chronic high dosage)

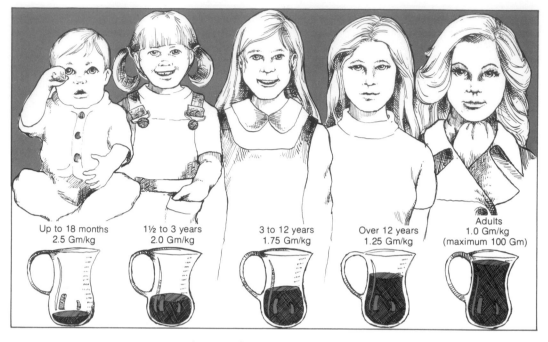

Up to 18 months
2.5 Gm/kg

1½ to 3 years
2.0 Gm/kg

3 to 12 years
1.75 Gm/kg

Over 12 years
1.25 Gm/kg

Adults
1.0 Gm/kg
(maximum 100 Gm)

How much glucose should you give?
The loading dose of oral glucose, usually a 25% solution, must be administered over several minutes in a dosage appropriate to the patient's age and body size.

obese patients). Usually, a 25% glucose solution flavored with noncaloric cola, orange, or lemon is given in the quantities shown in the above illustration.

At fasting, draw the antecubital venous blood specimen for adults or capillary blood for children. Note "time zero" when the patient starts drinking the glucose. Draw additional blood specimens exactly 60, 90, 120, and 180 minutes after time zero (and at 240 and 300 minutes after for a 5-hour test). In some cases, the physician may also order a 30-minute specimen on a patient.

You may also be asked to collect simultaneous urine specimens. Although not required for the interpretation of the test, they give information about the patient's renal glucose threshold, which is potentially useful in adjusting insulin dosage if such therapy is required.

If whole blood, without preservatives, is obtained, the specimens must be analyzed within a half hour after collection. So, you must deliver the specimens, properly labeled, promptly to the laboratory. Your laboratory may suggest that you collect the specimens in fluoride tubes, which make glucose assays valid for up to 48 hours.

If the patient vomits the ingested glucose during the first hour, the results will be invalidated, so you should cancel the test at once and re-schedule it for another day.

PATIENT'S INSTRUCTIONS FOR A GLUCOSE TOLERANCE TEST

Breakfast

Fruit or fruit juice	1 serving
Cereal	½ cup cooked or ¾ cup prepared
Bread	2 slices
Butter or margarine	1 tablespoon (2 pats) or 3 strips bacon
Cream	½ cup
Jelly or sugar	2 tablespoons

Dinner

Meat, fish, eggs, or cheese	1 average serving
Potato, rice, or macaroni	1 average serving
Cooked vegetable or salad	1 serving
Bread	2 slices
Dessert: pie, cake, pudding, ice cream, or fruit with cookies	1 average serving
Cream	3 tablespoons
Jelly or sugar	2 tablespoons
Butter or margarine	2 tablespoons

(A packed lunch may consist of two meat, cheese, or egg sandwiches, fruit, cake or cookies, and a candy bar.)

Supper

Meat, fish, eggs, or cheese	1 average serving
Potato, rice, or macaroni	1 average serving
Cooked vegetable or salad	1 serving
Bread	2 slices
Dessert: pie, cake, pudding, ice cream, or fruit with cookies	1 average serving
Jelly or sugar	2 tablespoons
Cream	3 tablespoons
Butter or margarine	2 tablespoons

One pint (2 cups) of milk is to be used during the day. Coffee and tea may be used as desired.

Diet is that recommended by Nutrition Clinic, University of Michigan Medical Center, Ann Arbor, Mich.

Preparing for your glucose tolerance test

1. Three full days before your glucose tolerance test, begin to follow the high-carbohydrate diet shown above. For the test results to be accurate, you must follow the diet as closely as possible, even if it means eating more than you usually do.

2. Avoid all alcoholic beverages (beer, wine, liquor) during the three days before the test.

3. During the 10 hours before the test, eat and drink *nothing* but water, and do not smoke.

4. Avoid physical and emotional stress during the 10 hours before the test.

5. Tell the doctor what drugs you are taking. Some may have to be discontinued before the test.

6. Other instructions:

_____
_____
_____
_____
_____
_____
_____
_____
_____

Glucose tolerance test curves
Glucose tolerance test curves for diabetic, latent diabetic, and normal adult patients. These curves do not apply to the elderly, in whom glucose tolerance is much higher.

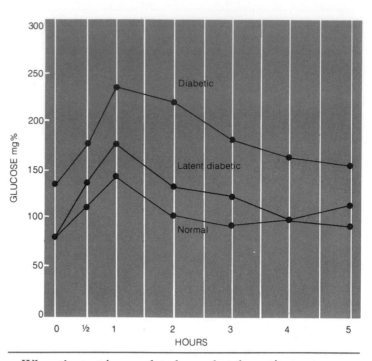

When the test is completed, see that the patient gets something to eat.

A variety of criteria for interpreting the test data are in use, and most results will fall in the clearly normal or clearly diabetic range. These criteria were established by various investigators so that patients could be classified as either diabetic or nondiabetic in various research protocols. But for the individual patient, such sharp classification is somewhat artificial, so the physician must judge his overall clinical condition to determine what follow-up or diagnosis is appropriate.

To interpret a patient's test results, you should know your hospital's normal values for the glucose tolerance test and whether the test was carried out and completed as planned. The above graph will help you to make a general interpretation of the test results.

Although the glucose tolerance test may be modified in several ways, these guidelines should help you obtain a reliable test — and set the stage for ongoing treatment with diet and perhaps oral hypoglycemic agents or insulin.

3

DIET: ENFORCING THE *SINE QUA NON*

BY SUSAN KAUFMANN, RN, BS

WHETHER A DIABETIC is adult onset or juvenile onset, severely diabetic or moderately diabetic, on insulin or on oral hypoglycemic agents...he's sure to need one type of therapy: Diet. Because diet is the *sine qua non* of diabetic therapy. After all, controlled intake of carbohydrates, fat, and protein — weighed against medications and exercise — keeps a patient balanced on that tightrope between hyperglycemia and hypoglycemia, diabetic coma and insulin shock.

Unfortunately, though, getting a diabetic patient to stick to a diet isn't simple. The usual litany of negatives that we give diabetic patients as a diet plan — "No desserts, no sugar in your coffee, no sporadic snacks" — hardly encourages cooperation. To encourage cooperation, you have to make the diet plan realistic for each patient's life-style. We've tried the realistic approach at the Joslin Clinic, and have found it often improves initial compliance. Of course, to guarantee continued compliance you've got to continue seeing each patient regularly and frequently. But a realistic diet-setting technique can help you handle the frustrations of initial diet instructions. The technique described in this chapter is based on our program, which applies primarily to adults. Chapter 14 suggests a few dietary modifications for diabetic children.

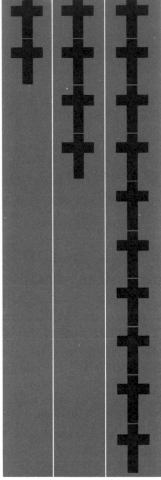

5-14% above ideal weight   15-24% above ideal weight   25% or more above ideal weight

The problem of fat
Being overweight jeopardizes the life of a diabetic. If he is 5 to 14% overweight, he runs twice the risk of mortality of a diabetic at ideal weight; 15 to 24% overweight, he runs four times the risk; and 25% or more overweight, he runs ten times the risk of death.

Tailoring objectives

Your therapeutic goals should be no different from those recommended by most textbooks. You should plan programs to help patients:
• reach and maintain ideal weight
• maintain proper nutrition
• assist in controlling their diabetes
• assist in preventing and controlling short-term and long-term complications.

The diet, though, should be tailored to the patient's specific life-style.

To really get to know each new patient and his life-style, we invite him for a week-long course at our diabetic treatment unit. Throughout the week, the unit's physicians give classes in the morning and we teaching nurses give classes in the afternoon. We encourage the patient to attend both sessions, and to come to us for private instruction to supplement or clarify classroom material. We also provide diet instruction both in class and individually. But the unit's dietitian embellishes on our instructions and consults patients with complicated dietary restrictions, such as gluten-free or lactose-free diets.

Throughout the week, we also ask the patient to critique his diet over and over, so we can modify it to make it realistic. In this way, he has some say in setting his dietary goals and maintaining his diabetic control. And by the end of the week, we're able to discharge him with a diet that he understands and that is tailored to his needs.

Begin where the patient is

To establish a dietary "starting point" during any instruction course, you should open by asking simple questions, "Why are you here? What would you like to know?"

If the patient says he's having difficulty with hypoglycemic episodes, begin there. Once you work out a dietary solution to that problem, you may go into gourmet meal planning — if that's what he wants. Your point, always, is to stress the *patient's* objectives, to gear your instruction to what *he* wants to know.

Early during your conversation, also determine the patient's life-style — his amount of activity, usual times of

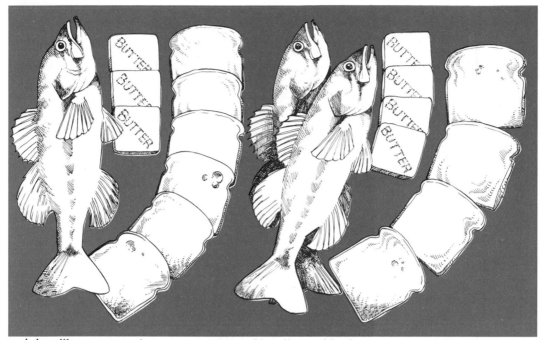

activity, illnesses or other stresses, type of insulin, and body response to insulin.

Then give him a "test" diet as a starting point.

You may follow the American Diabetes Association's diet (see page 210). But you may make some modifications. We base the actual number of calories that a patient requires on his ideal body weight and amount of activity:

20 calories per kg ideal weight =
                    caloric intake for weight loss
25 calories per kg ideal weight =
                    caloric intake for maintenance
30 calories per kg ideal weight =
                    caloric intake for increased
                    activity or weight gain.

The ADA suggests that 50% to 60% of these calories be consumed as carbohydrates, 10% to 15% as protein, and 30% to 35% as fat. But we generally stick to a 40-20-40 formula unless the patient has renal failure, elevated lipid levels, or other medical problems. We feel that patients don't tolerate the higher carbohydrate level as well as this lower level.

Our substitution list also resembles the ADA's exchange list, with four exceptions.

What's for dinner?
The diet of the American Diabetes Association recommends that 60% of all calories consumed be carbohydrates, 10% be protein, and 30% be fat. The Joslin Clinic diet observes the same categories in different quantities: 40-20-40. Check with the physician to see which diet is best for your patient.

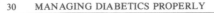

Understand CHO before giving them

In giving carbohydrates to prevent hypoglycemia or to treat insulin shock, remember the following analogy:

- sugar enters the blood as fast as a child runs;
- starch enters the blood as fast as a child walks;
- starch in vegetables enters the blood as fast as a child crawls.

To forestall hypoglycemia, you should suggest slower-acting starches for afternoon or evening snacks. To treat insulin shock, you should administer fast-acting sugars.

First, instead of one fruit list, we provide two — "small fruits" and "medium fruits." Small fruits can be interchanged with cookies, pretzels, and crackers; medium fruits can be interchanged with anything on the bread list.

Second, like the ADA we forbid concentrated sweets. But unlike the ADA we allow ice cream occasionally — at most once a week, unless there is some overriding reason for more, such as excessive exercise.

Third, we break down our vegetable list into "3%" and "6%" categories instead of using the ADA's vegetable categories. We think this terminology helps the patient remember the carbohydrate content of the vegetables — and reemphasizes the need to monitor intake of carbohydrates, protein, and fats.

Fourth, unless a patient is unusually inactive or the time between meals is unusually short, we generally don't recommend fruits for between-meal snacks. The reason is that we've found fruits metabolize quickly and don't always prevent hypoglycemia. Usually we suggest slowly metabolized carbohydrates, such as bread or crackers (see substitution chart on page 32), followed by a protein for more "staying power" such as a slice of cheese or peanut butter. Most patients on a single dose of intermediate-acting insulin (NPH) need only a midafternoon and evening snack, unless the time between breakfast and lunch is unusually long. More active patients generally need a midmorning snack too.

If we're working with a patient who frequents fast-food restaurants and snacks on "junk" food, we also give him a breakdown of the carbohydrate, protein, and fat content in these foods. (See snack and MacDonald's charts.)

Compromising for consistency

Does all this mean that, when a patient leaves your diet instruction course, he should leave with a rigid, written diet of basics and substitutions — and with the admonition to "stick to it"? No. You should give written instructions — tailored, of course, to the patient's individual needs (don't use preprinted form diets). But don't insist that he stick to it "or else."

Even though we devise a realistic diet plan for each patient, we realize that he may deviate from it. Some patients just can't break lifelong habits, even though they understand why they should; others find they can't restructure their daily lives to

NUTRIENT COMPOSITION OF GENERAL MILLS SNACKS

	Bows 100Gm	½oz	Bugles 100Gm	½oz	Buttons 100Gm	½oz	Daisy*s 100Gm	½oz	Whistles 100Gm	½oz
No. of pieces	152	22	104	15	339	48	198	28	120	17
Protein (Gm)	5.51	.8	5.63	.8	10.3	1.4	6.53	.9	9.28	1.3
Fat (Gm)	37.5	5.3	37.4	5.3	28.1	4	23.5	3.3	26.5	3.8
Carbohydrate (Gm)	52.5	7.5	52.5	7.5	54.7	7.8	61.8	8.8	56.1	8

NUTRIENT COMPOSITION OF MACDONALD'S FOODS

	Egg McMuffin 126.7 Gm	Hamburger 96.8 Gm	Cheeseburger 110.9 Gm	¼ lb. Hamburger 156.8 Gm	¼ lb. Cheeseburger 186.2 Gm	Big Mac 183.4 Gm
Protein(Gm)	17.6	13.0	16.1	26.5	31.4	26.2
Fat (Gm)	11.3	9.6	13.9	19.3	27.7	31.9
Carbohydrate (Gm)	35.2	27.8	30.0	33.4	36.3	41.2
Exchanges	2½ bread 1½ meat 1 fat	2 bread 1 meat 1 fat	2 bread 2 meat 1 fat	2 bread 3 meat 1 fat	2 bread 4 meat 2 fat	3 bread 3 meat 4 fat

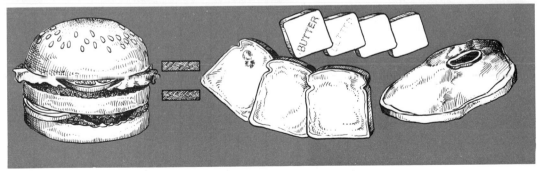

accommodate their discharge diet. So, we encourage each patient to keep in touch and to let us know if he encounters any problems with his diet. Our object, we assure patients, is to devise a diet they can live with.

Recently, for instance, Jan, a 19-year-old college student, came to the clinic for help with midafternoon insulin reactions.

Substitutions for 2 Uneeda biscuits plus ½ cup of whole milk

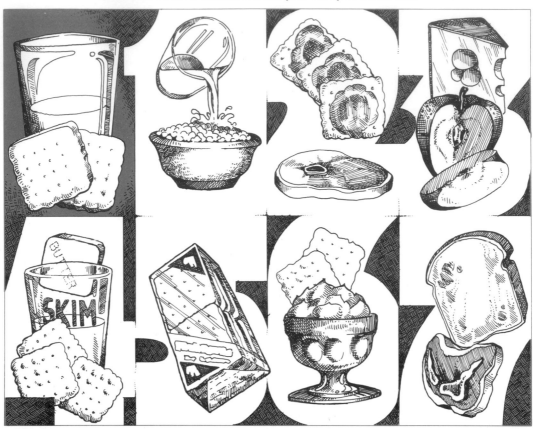

Substitutions for 2 Uneeda biscuits

FOOD	PORTION	FOOD	PORTION
Animal crackers	6	Veri-thin	2
Arrowroot biscuits	3	Veri-thin sticks	45
Brown Edge	2	Ritz or Cheese Ritz	5
Butter Thins	3	Rye Thins	6
Cheese Tidbits	20	Rye Krisp	2
Chocolate Snaps	4	Saltines	4 (2" x 2" each)
Ginger Snaps	3	Social Tea Biscuits	3
Graham Cracker	2 whole (2½" x 5")	Triangle Thins	10
Lemon Snaps	3	Triscuit	3
Lorna Doones	2	Vanilla Wafers — small	4
Oyster Crackers	20	Vegetable Thins	8
Pretzels (Nabisco Co.)		Waverly Wafers	4
Dutch	1	Wheat Thins	8
Pretzelettes	8	Zwieback	2
3-ring	4		

She was taking 50 units of NPH insulin and had a fasting blood sugar of 65 (normal nondiabetic range 60-100). Lowering her insulin to 40 units partially solved the problem, but when we took her diet history, we uncovered another problem. She never ate between meals. Her reason: "I don't want to gain weight."

Since Jan was very slender — in fact, underweight — we suggested that she eat a package of peanut butter Nabs in the afternoon. She firmly refused, saying she didn't want to add any calories to her diet. Rather than insisting she do it our way — and probably not having her cooperate — we redistributed her diet to provide the carbohydrate and protein coverage she needed in the afternoon. She cheerfully complied — and hasn't had midafternoon insulin reactions since.

In another case, George, a 27-year-old lawyer, consulted us for help planning his diets for camping trips. He liked backpacking and mountain climbing on weekends, but often experienced hypoglycemic symptoms in the afternoon. We explained that exercise tends to lower blood glucose levels and usually requires altering insulin, diet, or both. Since George managed his day-to-day 2800 calories diet (with 3 p.m. snack) well, our only recommendation was to increase his 3 p.m. snack during backpacking trips. In a few weeks, he returned complaining that the increased calories made him feel so full that he felt uncomfortable — and he still experienced hypoglycemic reactions in the afternoon. Our next suggestion: Reduce his insulin from 30 units of NPH to 20 units on the days he would be backpacking. He found that this adjustment, plus concentrated camp foods, solved his problem.

Both of these cases involved only minor compromises to solve medical problems. But sometimes you have to make major compromises simply to get a patient to adhere to a consistent diet. Insisting on an "ideal" diet with recalcitrant patients would be a waste of their time — and yours. Often, for instance, you must compromise on what you consider an adequate breakfast to get a patient to eat any breakfast at all. Or you must settle for a higher-than-recommended caloric intake to keep the patient on a consistent diet.

Oscar, for example, was far overweight at 310 pounds. So, our first diet plan included a hefty reduction in calories. As we outlined the plan to Oscar, we mentioned a daily sandwich, which is what he had told us he ate every lunch. Oscar balked.

Therapeutic treats

The top half of the opposite page shows a few acceptable substitutes for the recommended snack of 2 Uneeda biscuits (unsalted soda crackers) and ½ cup whole milk: ½ cup cereal with ½ cup whole milk, 3 Uneeda biscuits with 1 Tbsp. peanut butter or 1 oz meat, a medium fruit plus 1 oz cheese, 2 Uneedas plus 1 tsp butter and ½ cup skim milk, 4 peanut butter Nabs, 2 Uneedas plus ½ cup D-Zerta pudding, or 1 slice bread with 1 oz meat.

"One sandwich? That's all for lunch — every blessed day? I'll starve to death. Some days I need two sandwiches."

We started to explain the desirability of weight loss, but didn't get far. Clearly we were losing him. We backed down, and worked for something positive — consistency. To assure that his calorie intake would be the same every day, we added another sandwich at every day's lunch. But we insisted that he eat two sandwiches every day. Oscar agreed. He still has his large dimensions, but at least he maintains some semblance of diabetic control.

True, this method isn't ideal. And we don't claim to have solved the ongoing dilemma of getting diabetics to comply with their diets. But we've learned to approach dietary planning more positively and more realistically. And we're finding that that approach usually gets positive results with the initial diet. Of course, whether dietary controls must be supplemented with oral hypoglycemic agents or insulin depends on the patient's overall condition and the severity of his diabetes.

4

ORAL AGENTS: COMBATTING CONVENIENCE

BY GAIL B. ASKEW, Pharm D, AND
KENNETH I. LETCHER, Pharm D

FOR THE CHILD WHO DEVELOPS diabetes mellitus, diet and insulin are the only means of therapy. But for the adult-onset diabetic, there are two other alternatives: diet alone, or diet and oral hypoglycemic agents.

The advantage of oral therapy over insulin therapy is obvious: Convenience. But convenience also is the main disadvantage of oral therapy. Because without the daily inconvenience of an insulin injection, some patients underrate the gravity of their diabetes and slip off their prescribed diet and medication.

For just that reason, your role in oral therapy for diabetics isn't as limited as you might think. Many physicians who prescribe a hypoglycemic drug tell the patient to take it once or twice a day, and then send him out to manage his own therapy as best he can. In your contact with the patient, you have a tremendous opportunity to fill in what the doctor leaves out — explanations of how the drugs work, the risks, and how to keep those risks to a minimum.

Oral therapy isn't for everyone
For some diabetics, oral agents — the sulfonylureas, such as Orinase, and the biguanides, such as DBI — definitely have a place in treatment. They can't substitute for dietary controls. But as adjuncts to diet and as replacements for insulin injec-

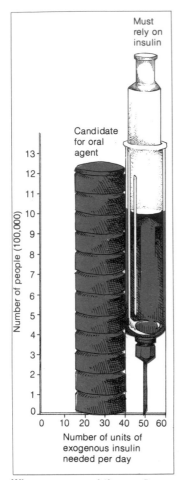

Must
rely on
insulin

Candidate
for oral
agent

13
12
11
10
9
8
7
6
5
4
3
2
1
0

Number of people (100,000)

0   10 20 30 40 50 60

Number of units of
exogenous insulin
needed per day

Who can use oral therapy?
A likely candidate for oral therapy
is the milder, nonketotic,
adult-onset diabetic. Control of
diet and exercise is just as
important as with
insulin-dependent patients,
perhaps more so since the
convenience of oral therapy may
cause the diabetic to
underestimate his condition.

tions, they do benefit many patients, medically and psychologically. Unfortunately, though, not all adult-onset diabetics are eligible for oral therapy.

Of all the criteria physicians use to select candidates, the most critical is pancreatic function.

The normal adult pancreas secretes 40 to 60 units of insulin each day, an amount that is essential for acceptable carbohydrate metabolism.

In overt diabetes, the pancreas secretes too little insulin. If a diabetic has no pancreatic function, he needs injections of 40 to 60 units of exogenous insulin each day to prevent hyperglycemia. If he has residual pancreatic function, however, he may be able to control his condition with dietary modifications and oral agents, since the oral agents regulate blood sugar using endogenous insulin. A good candidate for trial on oral hypoglycemics is a patient who would require less than 40 units of exogenous insulin per day, indicating some degree of pancreatic function.

The pancreatic function test generally rules out oral therapy for patients with juvenile-onset diabetes since they characteristically have no residual pancreatic function. Without pancreatic function, they're prone to life-threatening ketoacidosis as well as hyperglycemia. These patients need complete insulin replacement.

Patients with adult-onset diabetes, on the other hand, often have enough pancreatic function to produce some insulin and to resist ketoacidosis. They may be able to rely on oral hypoglycemic agents to regulate their blood sugar levels.

When we draw a profile of a likely candidate for oral therapy, we find that he has diabetes mellitus, is usually over 40 years old, is ketoacidosis-resistant, can't control his condition with diet alone, and needs less than 40 units of insulin per day. Of course, some other conditions, such as pregnancy or surgery, preclude oral therapy. The candidate must meet those criteria as well.

Even if the patient does meet all the criteria for oral therapy, though, the physician may place him on insulin. Why? Because the patient or his physician may decide that the risks of oral therapy outweigh its advantages. For example, some studies have implicated the oral hypoglycemics in a high incidence of cardiac deaths. Naturally, a diabetic with cardiac problems wouldn't want to risk further complications.

But if the physician does decide to try oral therapy, he must then make another decision: Whether to prescribe a sulfonylurea or biguanide.

The "undercover" agents

Many patients mistakenly believe that hypoglycemic agents are oral insulin. Nothing could be further from the truth; there is no such thing as oral insulin. If taken orally, insulin would be degraded and have no effect. Oral hypoglycemic agents are simply synthetic agents that help reduce blood sugar. Exactly how they regulate the blood sugar, though, is a matter of speculation.

Sulfonylureas seem to act primarily on the beta cells of the islets of Langerhans in the pancreas. These cells normally produce and secrete enough insulin to maintain the correct blood glucose level. As a person ages, though, these cells may become sluggish, impairing the body's response to rising blood glucose. Sulfonylureas initially stimulate the beta cells to release more insulin, thus lowering the blood glucose level.

After prolonged use, the sulfonylureas no longer cause an increase in insulin release. For some reason, however, the improvement in glucose tolerance is maintained. No one knows exactly why the sulfonylureas continue to work, but experiments suggest that the drugs may also increase glucose uptake in the peripheral tissues, resulting in decreased blood glucose levels.

A secondary function of the sulfonylureas involves the release of glucose from the liver. Normally, the liver and pancreas interact to maintain the blood glucose level. The liver stores glucose in the form of glycogen, which it reconverts to glucose and releases into the blood when needed to maintain the correct blood glucose level. To prevent the blood glucose from rising too high, the pancreas normally releases insulin. But in a diabetic, the pancreas can't release enough insulin to prevent hyperglycemia from the hepatic glucose release. By inhibiting the release of hepatic glucose, the sulfonylureas help balance the deficiency in pancreatic response.

The exact mechanism of action of the biguanides is not well understood. Animal and tissue studies have suggested several conflicting proposals. They all indicate, however, that in contrast to the sulfonylureas, the biguanides don't increase insulin secretion. In fact, although the biguanides can stabilize the blood sugar of diabetic patients, they have no hypoglycemic action in the nondiabetic. (For this reason, some doctors are

Barriers to oral therapy

Pregnancy. In addition to possibly causing teratogenic effects or congenital malformations in the fetus, oral agents may not control diabetes complicated by pregnancy. Furthermore, oral agents can cross the placental barrier, inducing hypoglycemia in the neonate; insulin can't.

Severe stress, surgery, fever, or infection. Any traumatic condition can trigger wide fluctuations in the patient's diabetic state, almost always demanding a temporary return to insulin therapy. Elderly patients are particularly prone to changes in response to their oral hypoglycemic agents, since their liver and renal functions may change markedly during illness.

Suspected "sulfa" allergy. Any previous allergic reaction to a sulfa drug bars sulfonylurea therapy, since the sulfonylureas are chemically related to the sulfonamide antimicrobial category of drugs.

A patient with a sulfa allergy can take biguanides, however, since they aren't chemically related to the sulfa drugs.

Predisposal to lactic acidosis. Although the biguanides don't actually cause lactic acidosis, they do seem to potentiate any tendency toward lactic acidosis that the patient may have.

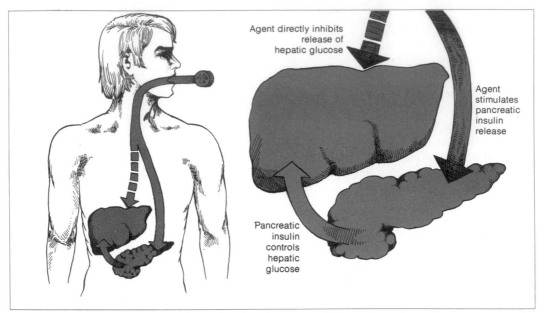

Agent directly inhibits release of hepatic glucose

Agent stimulates pancreatic insulin release

Pancreatic insulin controls hepatic glucose

How do sulfonylureas work?

To be effective, sulfonylureas require either insulin-producing beta-cells or the presence of some exogenous insulin. In receptive individuals they increase the manufacture and release of insulin in response to food and increase the glucose uptake in fat and in muscle. They may or may not decrease the secretion of glucagon, a pancreatic hormone that raises blood sugar levels. Under certain circumstances sulfonylureas may stimulate the formation of new beta-cells.

investigationally prescribing biguanides for patients with hyperinsulinism — or hypoglycemia. Although the FDA hasn't approved biguanides for this use, investigators report that biguanides seem to stabilize the blood sugar of these patients.)

One proposed mechanism of action for phenformin, the only biguanide available in the U.S., involves the increase in anaerobic glycolysis, which is the breakdown of glucose by non-air-dependent pathways. This results in lower blood glucose and a secondary increase in the peripheral utilization of glucose. It may also result in the severe problem of lactic acidosis, however.

Phenformin increases glucose uptake by clearing insulin from the general blood supply to the peripheral tissues. In contrast to the sulfonylureas, phenformin doesn't increase the blood insulin levels. In fact, it may decrease the release of insulin.

Another proposal suggests that phenformin controls hyperglycemia by impairing intestinal absorption of glucose, decreasing the total amount of glucose entering the blood. This enables the available endogenous insulin to control glucose levels. Phenformin also may decrease gluconeogenesis, which is the formation of glucose from protein or fat sources, thereby preventing an increase in the blood glucose level from that source.

COMPARISON OF ORAL HYPOGLYCEMICS

Generic name	Trade name	Dosage forms	Usual daily dose	Duration of action
Sulfonylureas tolbutamide	Orinase	500 mg	0.5-3 Gm usually in 3 divided doses	6-12 hrs.
tolazamide	Tolinase	100 mg 250 mg	0.1-1 Gm in 1 or 2 doses daily with meals (one with breakfast, second with evening meal if needed)	12-24 hrs.
acetohexamide	Dymelor	250 mg 500 mg	.25-1.5 Gm in 1 or 2 doses daily before meals (one before breakfast, second before evening meal if needed)	12-24 hrs.
chlorpropamide	Diabinese	100 mg 250 mg	0.1-0.5 Gm in 1 daily dose with breakfast	24-36 hrs.
Biguanides phenformin	DBI, Meltrol (tablet)	25 mg	0.025-0.15 Gm in 1 to 2 daily doses with meals	4-6 hrs.
	DBI-TD, Meltrol (capsule)	50 mg 100 mg	0.05-0.15 Gm in 1 or 2 doses daily with meals (one with breakfast, second with evening meal if needed)	12-14 hrs.

However the oral agents achieve their effects, all have a single goal: to regulate the blood sugar level. Naturally, though, the oral hypoglycemics do vary in duration of activity, dosages, and metabolism (see table). These elements influence the physician's choice of an oral hypoglycemic agent for a particular patient.

Chlorpropamide (Diabinese), which is excreted unchanged in the urine, is the longest acting oral agent. Since its effect may last as long as 36 hours, a patient usually has to take it only once a day.

Tolazamide (Tolinase) and *acetohexamide (Dymelor)* are intermediate-acting agents, which are metabolized in the liver. In fact, acetohexamide *must* be metabolized to be an active drug. The patient may be able to rely on once-a-day therapy with acetohexamide or tolazamide, although two daily doses may be necessary.

Tolbutamide (Orinase), also metabolized in the liver, is the shortest acting sulfonylurea. It must be taken two or three times a day to achieve a maximal effect.

Phenformin (DBI, DBI-TD, and Meltrol), the only biguanide available in the U.S., is relatively short-acting. Although it may be used alone, it is often used along with a sulfonylurea drug. Phenformin is used frequently for obese diabetics, since it doesn't increase the blood insulin levels. (An increase in insulin level would promote the transport of glu-

Canadian equivalents

In Canada, some names of oral hypoglycemic agents, particularly trade names, differ from the U.S. names. Here's a Canadian listing with the usual daily maintenance doses for each.

SULFONYLUREAS
acetohexamide: Dimelor (250 mg - 1.5 Gm)
chlorpropramide: Chloromide, Chloronase, Diabinase, Novopropramide, Stabinol (100 - 500 mgm)
glyburide: Euglucon (2.5 - 20 mg)
tolbutamide: Mobenol, Orinase, Tolbutone (0.5 - 3 Gm)

BIGUANIDES
metformin hydrochloride: Glucophage (1.5 - 4 Gm)

cose into fat tissues, thereby causing the patient to gain weight.) Because of its relatively short duration of action, a patient has to take phenformin tablets three times a day. It is also available in timed-disintegration capsules, though, which may decrease the frequency of administration to twice a day.

From this information, you can see that, for once-a-day convenience, chlorpropamide would be the drug of choice. Obviously, though, convenience isn't the only criterion for selection.

For example, one drawback of chlorpropamide is that it poses a greater risk of hypoglycemia since it is so long-acting. On the other hand, with short-acting agents, patients often forget to take the prescribed number of doses each day.

Preexisting renal or hepatic damage also plays an important role in the selection of the correct hypoglycemic. For example, it would be unwise to treat a diabetic with severe liver disease with any sulfonylurea other than chlorpropamide. All the other sulfonylureas undergo liver metabolism. (Acetohexamide must be metabolized to be active. Tolbutamide and tolazamide are metabolized to less active compounds for excretion; a decrease in liver metabolism could result in toxicity from either drug.) By the same token, caution should be taken with a diabetic with renal insufficiency using chlorpropamide or acetohexamide, since those drugs are excreted by the kidneys in an active form. Decreased kidney function would cause them to accumulate in the blood, leading to possible toxicity.

The choice of drug, however, is the doctor's responsibility. Yours is to make sure the patient understands the hows and whys of oral therapy, the pitfalls as well as the benefits.

Hard facts and caveats

Because they don't have to take an insulin injection every day, many patients on oral therapy tend to underrate the seriousness of their diabetes and the importance of treatment.

But the cold facts are that patients on oral therapy face risks, and complications just as insulin-dependent diabetics do. You must make a concerted effort to teach patients on oral therapy about dietary and drug management and about possible side effects.

For the patient on oral therapy, as for the insulin-dependent patient, the word *diet* goes hand in hand with diabetes. Indeed, for a patient on oral agents, diet plays a particularly crucial role, since he is relying on his endogenous insulin supply.

The physician will prescribe the patient's individual diet, selecting it according to his age, ideal weight, medical condition, activity, and eating habits. For the patient with overt diabetes, the physician will choose a diet from the ADA list (see Appendices), with a balanced level of carbohydrate, protein, and fat intake.

Whatever the diet selected for a particular patient, you should reinforce the physician's and dietitian's instructions, explaining the need for the balanced ratio of protein, carbohydrates, and fat. Be sure, too, to emphasize the "no cheating" rule, that effective therapy is based on the patient eating all prescribed foods. A rule of thumb for all diabetics: Undereating is just as hazardous as overeating.

Remind the patient that he may have to reduce his medication intake if he has a change in his level of physical activity, but that he should do so only with his doctor's approval. No self-prescribing.

To monitor the effects of diet, exercise, and medications on blood sugars, some doctors have their patients perform periodic urine tests, particularly during their first few weeks on therapy. Teaching them how to perform these tests will probably be your job. (See Chapters 6 and 7 for teaching instructions.) If the patient consistently gets very high or very low results, he should report them to his physician. The physician then may amend his dosage instructions, change the patient to another oral hypoglycemic agent or, in persistently severe cases, change the patient to insulin.

After the patient has been on oral therapy for a while and is well controlled, he may not have to test his urine except when he suspects adverse reactions.

You also should instruct patients on oral hypoglycemic therapy about foot care. Just like the insulin-dependent patient, the oral therapy patient is susceptible to foot infections and diabetic gangrene. Show him how to care for his feet just as you would show a patient on insulin (see Chapter 6).

After you've given these initial instructions to your patient, make sure he has understood them. Question him, or reverse roles and have him explain urine tests and diet and foot care to you. Even after you're sure he understands the instructions, follow up with periodic pep talks if possible.

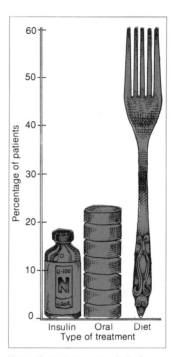

How diabetics control their condition
Most diabetics are able to control their condition by diet alone, an encouraging fact. Many patients combine methods, however, watching what they eat *and* taking insulin or oral hypoglycemics. Combinations are not represented in the above chart.

Oral hypoglycemics aren't for everyone
Thin adult-onset diabetics have responded less well to oral treatment than have overweight patients. In those who do respond well, however, blood glucose levels are more nearly normal than would be possible with insulin.

Perhaps the most helpful information you can give a diabetic on oral therapy is how to get the best mileage out of his medication with the least risk. The key is timing, both in the number of doses per day and the time of administration.

Frequency of administration depends on the particular agent, the patient's medical condition, and his response to therapy. Generally, the longest-acting agent, Diabinese, should be taken only once a day, in the morning. Drugs with shorter durations of action, such as tolbutamide, may be taken as often as two or three times a day. Find out the doctor's instructions and reinforce them.

Also impress your patient with two caveats of drug therapy.

First, if he is fasting for any reason — impending surgery or lab studies — he shouldn't take oral agents. Taking oral agents during fasting risks hypoglycemic reactions, since the glucose intake is decreased. In addition, the stress caused by the surgery or tests may cause fluctuations in the diabetic state, which may not be well controlled with the oral agents.

Second, he should not take his oral hypoglycemic at bedtime, unless he has a special order from his attending physician, since he could have a severe hypoglycemic reaction in his sleep. If you're caring for a diabetic on oral therapy in the hospital, don't give the oral agent at bedtime unless you're sure the order is valid. Have the order verified and notify your supervisor before giving the dose.

A rundown of risks
Both of these caveats underline an important point about oral therapy: Oral hypoglycemic agents are potent drugs, possibly even suicidal weapons, that must be treated with the same respect accorded to insulin. Both the biguanides and the sulfonylureas can produce dangerous side effects and adverse reactions.

Naturally, you don't want to frighten your patient by overemphasizing the risks of oral therapy. On the other hand, though, you don't want to treat the risks so casually that he ignores dietary precautions or handles his medication too carelessly. So, realistically explain adverse reactions; make sure your patient can recognize them in their incipient stages and can correct them swiftly. Also emphasize, though, that the risks are almost nil *if* he scrupulously follows his doctor's orders.

• *Hypoglycemia*. By far the greatest threat in sulfonylurea therapy is hypoglycemia, which curiously is the drug's therapeutic effect taken to extremes. Although hypoglycemia occurs infrequently with the sulfonylureas, it can cause severe illness, coma, or even death if it goes unrecognized and uncorrected. Hypoglycemia is rarely a threat to overt diabetics on biguanide therapy, however, since the biguanides don't stimulate insulin release.

Hypoglycemia can be precipitated by several conditions: changes in renal or hepatic function, fever, infection, surgery, or other stressful situations. For that reason, instruct your patient to call his doctor promptly at the first signs of illness. In cases of trauma or illness, the doctor may switch him temporarily to insulin therapy, since the insulin allows more individualized treatment.

Hypoglycemic effects of the sulfonylureas are potentiated by many drugs, including propranolol (Inderal), probenecid (Benemid), phenylbutazone (Azolid, Butazolidin), chloramphenicol (Chloromycetin), bishydroxycoumarol (Dicumarol), clofibrate (Atromid-S), sulfonamide-type antibacterial agents, and salicylates. Since aspirin can lower the blood sugar, be sure patients know to take Tylenol instead. Overdosage of oral hypoglycemics and undereating may also predispose a patient to hypoglycemia. List for the patient the early signs of hypoglycemic reactions: lethargy, sweating, hunger, inability to concentrate, shakiness, slight nervousness, irritability, dizziness, headaches, papitations, or tremors.

If a patient experiences any of these mild reactions, he can stem them quickly by simply eating any glucose-producing food — fruit juice, soft drinks, or candy. (See Chapter 11 for details on ways to stem hypoglycemia.) If his symptoms don't subside within 10 to 15 minutes, he should take another dose of candy or soft drinks and, if possible, test his urine. If symptoms still persist after 10 or 15 minutes and his urine proves negative, he should call his physician.

Although severe hypoglycemic reactions rarely occur with oral therapy, they can develop if mild reactions go untreated for a long period. Severe hypoglycemic reactions are characterized by grogginess, stupor, and unconsciousness. If the patient is simply groggy, a family member should place a spoon of honey or corn syrup in his mouth. His mucous membranes will absorb the substance, and the patient should

Scientific serendipity

The road to the discovery of oral hypoglycemics was paved with serendipity and accident. In 1942 Marcel Janbon, a Frenchman, was working with sulfa drugs to treat cases of typhoid when he found that one sulfa drug derivative (IPTD) lowered the blood sugar of his patients to the point of producing convulsions. Janbon's colleague, Auguste Loubatieres, began a prolonged series of animal studies to identify the cause. By 1955 Loubatieres had discovered that IPTD exerted no hypoglycemic effect in pancreatectomized animals. From this he deduced that the drug stimulated the pancreas to secrete insulin.

Neither Janbon nor Loubatieres explored the compound's usefulness in diabetes treatment. Instead Hans Franke and J. Fuchs, German scientists studying the hypoglycemic action of sulfa drugs, found that the antibacterial agent carbutamide lowered blood sugar. They demonstrated its usefulness in the treatment of diabetes and soon after the first oral hypoglycemic was introduced.

revive enough to drink a glass of fruit juice. If the patient becomes unconscious, however, he should be taken to a hospital emergency room, where he probably will require I.V. glucose.

● *Lactic acidosis.* Numerous cases of lactic acidosis have been reported in phenformin-treated patients. All of the cases, however, involved patients who were predisposed to lactic acidosis by their other medical problems. Some doctors now question the claim that phenformin can cause lactic acidosis. Still, you and your patient should watch out for it, since it's a severe condition associated with a high mortality rate.

Several medical conditions will predispose a patient to lactic acidosis. It can result from ischemia due to sustained hypotension, which may be present in hemorrhage, septicemia, shock, or heart failure. It also can result from renal insufficiency, starvation, and pregnancy. Take special care with phenformin patients who develop or already have any of these conditions.

Early clinical symptoms of lactic acidosis include hyperventilation and acute changes in the state of consciousness. Many people mistake lactic acidosis for ketoacidosis, since the clinical pictures are nearly the same. Lactic acidosis can be confirmed by laboratory tests showing elevated serum lactate with a low serum bicarbonate.

● Any marked change in consciousness indicates the need for rapid medical attention. The correct diagnosis for the cause of the change in mental state is essential.

● *Hyperglycemia.* Naturally if a patient forgets to take his medication regularly, he can have a return of his initial symptoms of hyperglycemia. He also may be more prone to hyperglycemia if he is taking thiazide diuretics, which aggravate the diabetic state and may increase requirements for oral agents. Symptoms of hyperglycemia, usually vague and mild at first, include loss of appetite, lethargy, nausea, vomiting, a high urine sugar, positive urine acetone reading, frequent urination, and marked thirst. If untreated for a prolonged period, the patient eventually could go into a diabetic coma.

The best way to ward off hyperglycemia, of course, is to follow dietary and drug instructions. A patient with mild symptoms usually can correct them by returning to his prescribed regimen. For persistent, severe symptoms, however, the patient should be seen by his physician; he may require insulin and fluid replacement therapy to correct the hyperglycemia.

● *Alcohol intolerance*. One side effect of the sulfonylureas is an Antabuse-like reaction, which may occur when a patient drinks alcoholic beverages. In fact, the patient may actually appear drunk — stumbling, slurring his words, having trouble remembering. He also may be flushed, nauseated, and tachycardic. Although alcohol intolerance usually is mild, it can cause severe headaches and vomiting and can produce symptoms lasting up to one hour.

The best cure for this reaction is the avoidance of alcohol. Warn your patient to be careful when he drinks. If your patient experiences any symptoms of alcohol intolerance, he should eliminate his drinking.

● *Drug incompatibilities*. In addition to drugs that potentiate the effects of the sulfonylureas, there are other types of drugs that interact with the sulfonylureas. Barbiturates, sedatives, and hypnotics may have a significantly prolonged effect in a patient taking sulfonylureas. The combination of methyldopa (Aldomet) and the sulfonylureas may produce blood dyscrasias. Both sulfonylureas and the phenothiazine tranquilizers can cause jaundice or abnormal results in liver function tests; taken together, they might produce a significant change in liver function. Although the patient's physician will take these interactions into account when he prescribes oral agents, this information may help you assess the patient's condition in an emergency situation.

Just for reference, you also should know that the sulfonylureas alone can produce a host of side effects: anorexia, nausea, vomiting, diarrhea, blood dyscrasias, hemolytic anemia, and allergic skin reactions (usually transient). Gastrointestinal irritation is the most common side effect, and may call for a reduction in dose or the use of divided drug therapy.

Phenformin has fewer reported side effects: mainly, gastrointestinal upsets and anorexia. Many patients on phenformin also have reported a metallic taste, which usually signals the maximum tolerable dose. The physician should be notified, so that a slight reduction in dosage can be made. By reducing the dose, the doctor can usually eliminate the taste while maintaining good diabetic control.

Serious side effects are rare, but they should be reported

SOME ACTIONS OF INSULIN, SULFONYLUREAS, AND PHENFORMIN			
	Insulin	Sulfonylureas	Phenformin
MAJOR ACTION	Increased glucose transfer into cells	Increased insulin secretion	Increased anaerobiosis
SUBSIDIARY EFFECTS: Insulin secretion	Decreased	Increased	Decreased
Glucose uptake by peripheral tissues	Increased	Increased	Increased
Blood-sugar lowering effect Normal subjects Depancreatized subjects	Marked Marked	Moderate None	None Slight
Marked hypoglycemia	Common	Rare	None
Lactate utilization	Increased	Increased	Decreased
Irreversible side effects	Present	Rare	None

immediately to the physician. Sometimes the side effects can be easily corrected by adjusting the dosage or by switching to another hypoglycemic agent or insulin.

A patient on oral therapy may complain of headaches and weakness a couple of hours after eating. These symptoms could mean that the patient needs a smaller dose of his drug or that his diet is not balanced. If he complains of these symptoms, have him record his food intake. You may be able to eliminate the symptoms simply by adjusting his diet or urging him to stick to it more closely. If the symptoms persist, report them to the physician.

Two different outcomes
How well does oral therapy work for patients? Should you take particular precautions with particular patients? Is oral therapy always successful? The following examples may help answer those questions.

Mildred, a wiry 40-year-old, had an almost classic case of adult-onset diabetes mellitus, discovered in an almost classic way. For several months she had seemed a different person, snapping at her colleagues at work for no apparent reason and feeling constantly irritable. Her concentration also slipped, she often broke into tears at the slightest provocation, and she constantly felt exhausted, thirsty, and hungry. Even though she snacked every couple of hours, her hunger and thirst persisted and she began losing weight.

For a while, she accepted the opinion of sympathetic friends who said it was "change of life." But when she began having to struggle to keep her weight up, she finally consulted a physician. He promptly sent her to the hospital for a workup, including a fasting blood sugar test. The test showed an abnormally high level, 160 mg/100 ml, so the physician ordered a 2-hour postprandial blood glucose, which also was elevated at 170 mg/100 ml.

Mildred's physician started her on Dymelor at a standard dose of 250 mg twice a day, before breakfast and before dinner. Within a few days, Mildred began to feel like herself again. And within a week or so she was completely rid of her insatiable hunger. In fact, she felt so good that, like many new diabetics, she often forgot to take her pills.

When Mildred returned to the doctor's office, complaining again of her earlier symptoms, the nurse explained diabetes to her. She emphasized that oral therapy is not a cure but rather a way to avert serious problems now and in the future. But, she said, it could be effective only if Mildred followed the prescribed regimen to the letter. She showed her how to keep a chart of her daily medications. And she stressed that her role was simply that of an advising nurse, not a nursemaid; Mildred would have to take full custody of her own daily care.

With these explanations, Mildred was soon back on her therapy schedule. Now, more than 3 years after she began therapy, she is still successfully managing her condition with Dymelor.

Unfortunately, though, not all patients have such success. Some may not be able to take oral agents from the start (primary failure); others start off well on them and then, for some unknown reason, the drugs seem to lose their effectiveness (secondary failure). Steve, for example, discovered his diabetes when he came into the hospital for a hernia repair. Tests showed his fasting blood sugar to be 180 mg/100 ml and consistently elevated levels in his glucose tolerance.

At first the physicians placed Steve on insulin therapy in the hospital, since his surgery, minor as it was, caused his diabetic state to fluctuate considerably. Just before he was discharged, though, they switched him to Orinase, 500 mg, twice a day. Steve left the hospital. Within a week, he was back with a blood sugar level just as high as it had been before. After a long talk with him, the nurse was convinced that he had been taking his pills and hadn't been cheating on his diet. The doctor slowly increased Steve's Orinase dose to the recommended maximum of 3 Gm daily.

When Steve's diabetes was not controlled at that dose, the physician added Meltrol to his drug regimen. Steve's condition didn't stabilize. The physician then increased the Meltrol to the maximum dose of 150 mg daily, with the Orinase at 3 Gm, but Steve's condition still failed to respond. At that point the physician decided that Steve's condition just couldn't be controlled with oral therapy. He switched him again, this time to Lente insulin. Within a few days, Steve's condition stabilized.

No one knows why patients like Steve don't succeed on oral therapy. Some have even been able to get along on as little as 18 units of insulin a day (a dose that indicates fairly strong pancreatic functioning) but still can't rely on oral medications. Fortunately, though, these patients are the exception rather than the rule. Diabetic patients who do benefit from their oral hypoglycemic therapy, both psychologically and medically, deserve the opportunity to use that treatment. You can provide them with a much needed service by remembering that they are still diabetics, and by teaching and encouraging them accordingly.

5

INSULIN: EASING THE DAILY ROUTINE

BY LAWRENCE W. WOLFE, BSc, RPh

JUST BECAUSE insulin therapy becomes a daily routine for some diabetics, don't think it's simple. Even nurses in hospitals make mistakes in insulin therapy — mismatching concentrations and syringes, confusing the different types of insulin, ignoring the best injection time for short-acting and long-acting insulins, even neglecting to rotate injection sites.

You could hardly call it child's play. Yet ironically it's life-saving therapy for about 200,000 children — and more than 1 million adults who can't control their disease with diet and oral agents. As with oral or dietary therapy, you'll probably be the person responsible for teaching patients both the practices and pitfalls of this therapy. How can you do that without fully understanding it yourself? Obviously, you can't. You must know how insulin works and how insulin therapy can be adapted to each patient's needs.

Just what is insulin?

As explained in Chapter 1, insulin is a major anabolic hormone that regulates carbohydrate, fat, and protein metabolism. It acts primarily in the liver, adipose tissue, and muscle to promote glucose uptake, stimulate glycogen synthesis, and suppress glucose production. When a patient's body fails to produce enough insulin, the patient has to control his glucose

TABLE 1 — TYPES OF INSULIN					
	ONSET (MIN)	PEAK (HRS)	DURATION	PH	INSULIN APPEARANCE
Short-acting					
Regular (NRL)	20-30 min	3-5 hrs	5-8 hrs	7-4	clear
Semilente	30-45 min	4-6 hrs	12-16 hrs	neutral	cloudy
Intermediate					
Globin	2-4 hrs	6-8 hrs	12-18 hrs	acid	clear
NPH	60-90 min	8-12 hrs	24-28 hrs	neutral	cloudy
Lente	60-90 min	8-12 hrs	24-28 hrs	neutral	cloudy
Long-acting					
PZI	3-6 hrs	14-20 hrs	36+ hrs	neutral	cloudy
Ultralente	5-8 hrs	16-18 hrs	36+ hrs	neutral	cloudy

Canadian equivalents

Generally, names of the various insulins are the same in Canada as in the U.S. There are two differences, though: Canada doesn't have Globin insulin, and it does have Sulfated insulin for insulin-resistant diabetics who need more than 200 units daily. (With Sulfated insulin, these patients can manage their diabetes on 1/10 to 1/5 their previous dose.) Also U-500 isn't available in Canada.

intake through diet and may have to either stimulate insulin production with oral agents or supplement his endogenous insulin with injections of exogenous (beef or pork) insulin.

Unfortunately, many nurses fail to explain the variations in the types and concentrations of insulin when they teach insulin therapy to new diabetics. Perhaps they assume that a patient would only become confused by an "information overload" about medications he won't be taking. On the contrary, I have found that many patients become confused by a *lack* of information. Without understanding the variables in insulin therapy, they may use the wrong syringe with their insulin, mistime their injections, or skip doses.

There are, of course, several types of insulin. These fall into three general categories: short-acting (quick uptake and short duration — Regular and Semilente), intermediate (Globin, NPH, and Lente), and long-acting (slow uptake and long duration — PZI and Ultralente).

Within these categories, each type of insulin has its own onset, peak, and duration of action (see Table 1). The variety in action, coupled with varieties in concentrations and doses, allows a physician to tailor insulin therapy to each patient's highly individual needs. (You'll notice that NPH and Lente have about the same onset and duration of action. However, they differ in basic makeup. NPH insulin contains zinc and two proteins — protamine and globin — to prolong its action. By utilizing 10 times more zinc, Lente — composed of Semilente and Ultralente — achieves the same duration without any foreign modifying protein. So it can be used by patients who are allergic to the proteins in NPH).

Each type of insulin comes in three concentrations: U-40, U-80, and U-100.

These terms refer to the concentration of insulin per milliliter of liquid — 40 units per ml, 80 units per ml, and 100 units per ml. Each concentration of insulin comes with its own syringe, specially calibrated for that concentration only. One of the leading causes of dosage errors in insulin therapy is mismatching syringe and concentration. If a patient should have 20 units of U-100 insulin and he or the nurse gives U-100 insulin in a U-40 syringe, for example, the dose will be more than twice the prescribed amount. Or if the patient should have 20 units of U-40 insulin and he or the nurse gives it in a U-100 syringe, the dose will be less than half the prescribed one.

Eventually U-100 insulin, which was introduced about three years ago, will replace U-40 and U-80 insulins. With a standard concentration, patients probably will make far fewer dosage errors.

All U-100 insulin today is "single-peak" — a highly purified product containing approximately 90% insulin and 9% insulin-like substances. Older products contained only 92% of these components and caused far more antigenicity. (Single-component insulin, which is 99% pure insulin, isn't available in the U.S. because it's considerably more expensive yet is only slightly more beneficial than single-peak insulin).

U-500 insulin also is available for treatment of coma and cases of insulin resistance requiring large doses of insulin.

Table 1 summarizes the onset, peak, and duration of each type of insulin based on the average person's response. But not all patients are "average." Some may respond differently, depending on several conditions:

• *Route of administration.* Most insulins must be given subcutaneously; only Regular insulin may be given intravenously. (If given subcutaneously, Regular insulin's onset and peak are delayed and its duration prolonged.) Insulin can be given intramuscularly for a faster onset in emergencies but the onset with I.M. administration can be unpredictable, so most doctors prefer I.V. administration.

• *Vascularity of the injection site.* Commonly used injection sites, such as the upper arms, thighs, and stomach, have a high degree of vascularity, which prompts absorption of insulin. Absorption will slow if the patient's vascular system is impaired — say, from muscular atrophy, edema, renal disease, or some systemic diseases.

• *Physical changes in the insulin.* These include chemical deterioration and contamination by other types of insulin.

• *Concentration.* As concentration increases, so does the duration of the insulin effect.

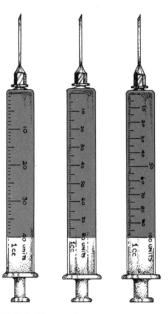

Match, then mix
Tell your patient to make sure he's using the correct syringe for his insulin. The syringe on the left, used only for U-40 insulin (40 units of insulin in 1 cc), is scaled red. The middle syringe, scaled in green, is used only for U-80. The syringe on the right, scaled in black, is especially suited for the new U-100 insulin.

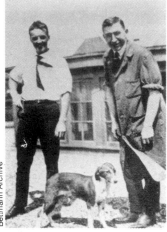

Bettmann Archive

Bad practice brings good luck
In 1920 Frederick Banting's practice as an orthopedic surgeon was slow. Because he had lots of spare time, he happened across an account of an 1889 experiment by Oskar Minkowski and Joseph von Mering. They had been studying the digestive function of the pancreas, and by accident they found that pancreatectomized dogs exhibit metabolic aberrations similar to those seen in human diabetics. This gave Banting ideas.

He decided to isolate from the pancreas the substance that could lower blood sugar. Working with Charles H. Best, a college senior, he discovered "isletin" (later named insulin), which quickly and effectively lowered blood sugar in a diabetic dog. The first human to try the new discovery was Leonard Thompson, age 14, whose diabetes had been ineffectively maintained, in the popular manner of the time, with a daily diet of 450 calories. Emaciated, lethargic, and near death, Thompson volunteered for treatment. His improvement was immediate and dramatic.

• *Biological and physiological variations.* Different patients may respond differently to the same dose of insulin.

Patients should know that any of the above conditions could affect their response to insulin and that they should contact their doctor for a change in dose.

Timing and storing, mixing and matching

Just as important as getting the right insulin in the right concentration, dose, and syringe is taking it at the right time. Patients don't need an intricate timetable for each individual type of insulin, but they should understand the rationale for timing doses.

Generally, patients on short-acting insulin should take it about 30 minutes before meals. Since it begins working within 20-45 minutes, this timing will ensure enough glucose intake at onset to prevent hyperinsulinism. All intermediate and long-acting insulins should be taken about 1 hour before meals. That will allow a leeway for their delayed onset.

Preparation for injection really begins with storage of the insulin bottle. All insulin will remain potent up to 36 months in a refrigerator and up to 18-24 months at room temperature (68-70°). At high temperatures (around 100°), insulin loses its potency within a couple of months; when frozen, it remains potent but the insulin may collect in tiny clumps, making withdrawal of a uniform dose difficult. Generally, though, a patient shouldn't worry about potency if he uses his common sense in storing his insulin. As long as he avoids leaving it in the glove compartment of a hot car or on the shelf during a long hot spell, the insulin should remain stable until the expiration date marked on the label.

If a patient is unsure about the potency of a bottle of insulin, though, he can easily check it by examining its color. Regular and Globin insulin should be clear; others should be cloudy and free of clumps or aggregations. If they don't meet these requirements, he should discard the bottle.

The patient should know, too, not to draw up his insulin hours in advance and leave it stored in the syringe. Insulin has a tendency to cling to glass and plastic if left in syringes, so he might not get an adequate dose. He also shouldn't inject insulin if it's cold. The coldness might delay absorption and could set off a local reaction.

Chapter 6 graphically shows the proper techniques for draw-

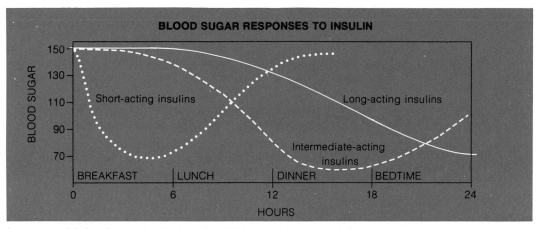

BLOOD SUGAR RESPONSES TO INSULIN

BLOOD SUGAR

150
130
110
90
70

Short-acting insulins

Long-acting insulins

Intermediate-acting insulins

BREAKFAST | LUNCH | DINNER | BEDTIME

0   6   12   18   24

HOURS

ing up and injecting a single insulin. If the patient must mix Regular insulin with a modified insulin, he should first make sure both are the same concentration. Then he should follow stringent guidelines for mixing insulins. If he should take, say, 15 units of NPH and 5 units of Regular insulin, he would follow this protocol:

• Observing aseptic precautions, inject 5 units of air into the bottle of Regular insulin and withdraw the needle.

• Inject 15 units of air into the NPH bottle and withdraw 15 units of insulin. Eliminate all air bubbles from the barrel of the syringe and the hub of the needle.

• Insert the needle into the bottle of Regular insulin, making sure the needle doesn't rest in the air space above the fluid. Withdraw 5 units of Regular insulin. (By injecting 5 units of air into the Regular bottle during the first step, the patient creates positive pressure within the bottle. This prevents the NPH in the syringe from leaking into the bottle and contaminating the Regular insulin.)

Some doctors may prefer that you tell the patient to reverse the order of these guidelines — that is, that he draw up the Regular insulin first and the NPH insulin second. Whatever the case, be sure the patient understands that he must use the same procedure every day — both at home and in the hospital. This will avoid any serious problems with so-called "dead space."

Dead space refers to that area in the tip of the syringe and in the hub and shaft of the needle where insulin remains after an injection is given. If a patient is taking a single dose of insulin and is careful to remove any air bubbles that could displace this residual or "dead" insulin, dead space won't present any problems. But if he must mix insulins, it can skew his dosages.

Blood sugar responses to insulin
You can see why physicians prescribe insulin with different lengths of action. They keep the patient's blood sugar well within normal limits because they peak at different times.

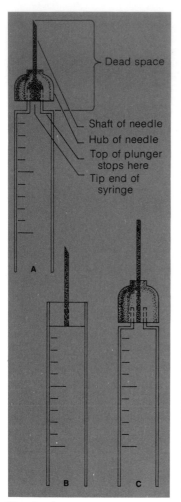

The dead space trap
A. In this model the space between the end of the plunger and the beginning of the needle (dead space) is considerable.
B. Because the top of the plunger stops where the needle begins, the only dead space in this syringe is inside the needle itself.
C. Although this model has a detachable hub, the needle shaft ends just above the top of the plunger. As a result, there is almost no dead space.

Because the two insulins mix in the syringe, the residual insulin will be subtracted from his prescribed doses.

Let's say, for example, that a patient is using a syringe with a dead space of 0.1 cc (10 units of U-100 insulin). The patient should take 6 units of Regular insulin and 50 units of NPH insulin. If he draws up the Regular insulin first, he'll get 16 units of it (10 units in the dead space and 6 in the syringe). When he adds 50 units of NPH insulin, the two will mix. And when he gives himself an injection, he'll get only part of the NPH insulin plus a little extra Regular insulin (42 units of NPH and 14 units of Regular). If he reverses the order of drawing up, though, he'll draw up 60 units of NPH insulin and 6 units of Regular insulin. Then, when he gives his injection, he'll get about 51 units of NPH and only 5 units of Regular insulin.

If the patient sticks to one order of drawing up, he can make any necessary adjustments in dosage and control his diabetes. But if he switches back and forth, he'll get fluctuating doses; control will be almost impossible.

No matter how carefully a doctor calculates a patient's insulin dose, chances are he'll have to modify it periodically to adapt to changes in the patient's health and life-style. Each patient should check his urine regularly, as he would with oral hypoglycemic agents, to assess his changing needs. If he is on a short-acting insulin and spills a lot of sugar in his urine between breakfast and lunch, he probably should increase his insulin dose by 2 units. But if his urine sugar is low before lunch, he should probably decrease his dose by 4 units. If the patient is on an intermediate insulin and spills a lot of sugar in his urine in the late afternoon and evening, he should probably increase his dose by 2 units. But if his urine sugar is low in late afternoon and evening, he probably should decrease his dose by 4 units. If the patient is on a long-acting insulin and his urine sugar is low in the morning, he probably should reduce his dose.

In addition to these adjustments, a patient may have to change his insulin dose during periods of extreme stress or exercise. Unless his doctor has authorized him to make dosage adjustments himself, though, he should consult his doctor before making any changes.

Hazards remain, local reactions wane
The hazards of diabetes — neuropathies, ketoacidosis, and so

EFFECTS OF DEAD SPACE AND ORDER OF MIXING ON INSULIN DOSAGE					
	Doctor's order	Using a syringe with 0.1 cc dead space, and drawing up the Regular insulin first	Using a syringe with 0.1 cc dead space, and drawing up the NPH insulin first	Using a syringe with 0.05 cc dead space, and drawing up the Regular insulin first	Using a syringe with no dead space
NPH insulin	50 units	42 units	51 units	46 units	50 units
Regular insulin	6 units	14 units	5 units	10 units	6 units

forth — threaten a patient on insulin as they do patients on oral hypoglycemic agents or diet alone. In fact, in some cases they threaten the insulin patient more because his condition is more severe. Still, with careful adherence to therapy, and with daily precautions such as foot care, patients can minimize the threats.

Coming chapters will thoroughly discuss the most serious systemic reactions to insulin therapy — insulin-induced shock and HHNK — as well as the ever-present threat of keto-acidosis. But here let's talk about less serious but equally important local reactions.

Some patients, particularly young women, suffer from facial edema and sometimes edema of the extremities from insulin injections. This usually subsides within a couple of days. If not, the doctor may prescribe a low-salt diet and a mild diuretic. About 30% of all patients develop painful edema around the injection site, which also subsides within a couple of days.

Fortunately the advent of single-peak (purified) insulin has cut the incidence of these reactions. But you should forewarn patients so they don't become overly concerned if they experience them.

A small percentage of patients develop fatty atrophy at injection sites. Although dimpling usually is minor, some patients may develop crater-like cavities measuring 4-5 inches in diameter and up to 3 inches deep. Usually, though, rotation of injection sites will prevent such serious complications.

Insulin therapy certainly isn't simple. But with the above instructions, most patients — even young children — will soon be managing it with few difficulties.

SKILLCHECK 1

1. Morton O'Reilly, a 40-year-old executive, has been admitted to the CCU because of acute chest pain. After 3 days, he is scheduled for discharge because neither his EKG nor cardiac enzymes shows evidence of a myocardial infarction. During hospitalization, though, Mr. O'Reilly has had several fasting blood sugar tests that showed moderate elevation. Should he have a glucose tolerance test before being sent home? Why?

2. Willard Jones is an 85-year-old resident of a nursing home. During a routine physical examination, his blood chemistry profile (fasting) shows his blood sugar to be 130 mg/dl. Do you think he should have a GTT?

3. Martha Simon, a 27-year-old salesclerk, takes 4 units of Regular insulin and 26 units of NPH insulin every morning. She eats breakfast at 7 a.m. and lunch at noon. On very active days, though, she frequently experiences hypoglycemic reactions around 10 a.m. What would you suggest to alleviate her hypoglycemic episodes?

4. Sixteen-year-old Julie takes 8 units of Regular insulin and 38 units of NPH. She tries to follow her diet but finds that even when she does, her bedtime Clinitest reads 2%. To compound matters, Julie frequently has hypoglycemic reactions during the night. She has tried to alleviate them by eating a piece of fruit before bed, but this doesn't seem to help. She says she doesn't want to increase her caloric intake by increasing her diet. What could you suggest to Julie?

5. Paul, age 14, is always hungry and eats continuously. He takes 50 units of Lente insulin and has been given a 3200-calorie diet appropriate to his age, size, and activity. Paul says that all his urine tests read 2% but he can't stop eating and needs huge quantities of food. What alternatives would you investigate?

6. Harold Jefferson, a 52-year-old accountant with a history of hypertension and congestive heart failure, has just been diagnosed as diabetic. He has been taking digoxin (Lanoxin) and hydrochlorothiazide (HydroDIURIL) for his other medical conditions: he is allergic to sulfisoxazole (Gantrisin). Would you expect the doctor to place Mr. Jefferson on oral hypoglycemic agents? Would any of the oral agents be more acceptable than others? Why?

7. Jane Scarlotti, a 43-year-old mother, manages her diabetes well with phenformin and diet. Her urine tests record between 1+ and 0 and she says she feels fine except for one thing: Her mouth always tastes like paper clips, even when she uses toothpaste and mouthwashes. She says she'll have to get breath mints to overcome the taste. Would you be concerned about the funny taste? How would you recommend that Mrs. Scarlotti cure her problem?

8. Sarah Steinman, a 39-year-old newly diagnosed diabetic, has been told to take 42 units of NPH insulin and 7 units of Regular insulin. After two weeks, she reports wild fluctuations in response to her therapy; some days she has hypoglycemic reactions and other days she feels fine. When she describes her injection technique, it sounds fine. What are some likely causes of the fluctuations?

9. Six months after beginning therapy on oral hypoglycemic agents, Frank Fisher is hospitalized with congestive heart failure. A new nursing student notices that Mr. Fisher has diabetes and is being treated with phenformin at home. She asks you why his phenformin hasn't been ordered in the hospital to maintain control. What explanation would you give her? Would Mr. Fisher's phenformin therapy be cause for concern in light of his congestive heart failure? Why?

10. Jacqueline Bond is a "Type A," competitive personality with a responsible job. She takes 44 units of Lente insulin once daily. Although she eats a fairly standard meal for breakfast and dinner, Ms. Bond's lunches vary from nothing at all to a full-course meal with cocktails. She feels that the large lunches are necessary for business. How would you advise Ms. Bond to change her eating habits?

HOW TO
INSTRUCT PATIENTS

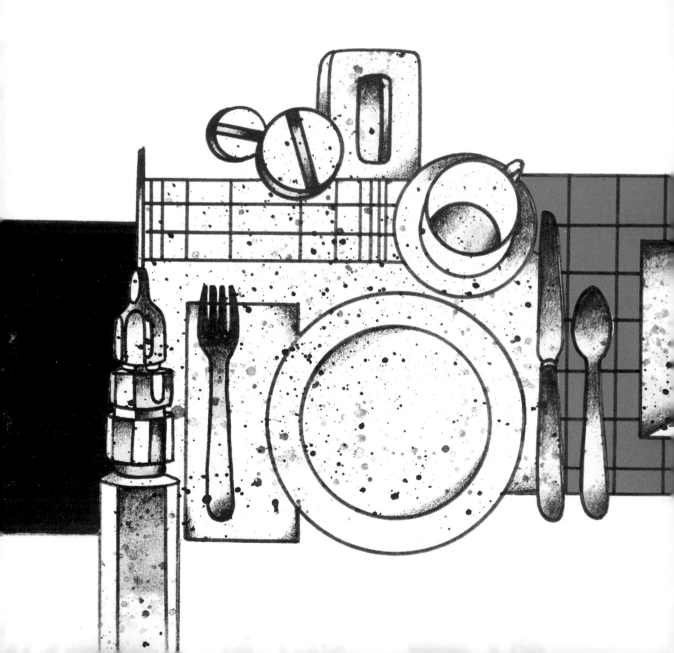

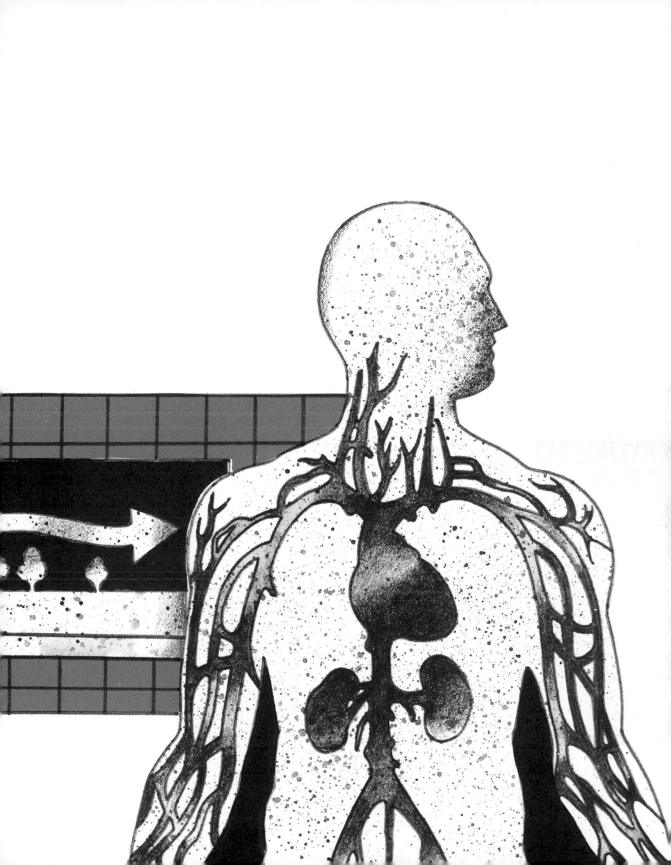

6

TURNING A PATIENT INTO A MANAGER

BY VERONICA ENGLE, RN

FEW DISEASES DEMAND as much patient participation in therapy as diabetes does. In fact, nearly all diabetics must manage their disease by themselves in everyday life. That may relieve you of the responsibility for managing therapy. But it also places a perhaps even more difficult responsibility on you — making the patient a knowledgeable, willing manager of his own care.

Many diabetes education programs rely heavily on pre-printed materials that aren't individualized, are difficult to read, and are confusing. This chapter, however, presents *basic* patient education material. In addition to showing the patient these, you should give him some handouts that repeat all instructions. Not only will these reinforce what you have taught him; they will also provide him with a handy reference at home. Following are two handout suggestions.

● *Diabetes and You*. A pamphlet, suitable for both insulin-dependent and non-insulin dependent patients, that would compare the human body to a car. As instructor, you would explain that both require fuel (gasoline or food), but to burn the fuel, both need a starter (key or insulin). Use the word "food" rather than "carbohydrate" to emphasize the importance of the total diet. You could use the car analogy to point out the

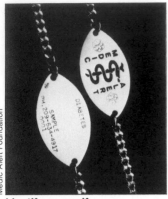

Identify yourself
It is important for diabetics to carry some kind of identification such as these Medic Alert bracelets so that in an emergency their condition will be treated properly.

patient's responsibility in self-care (just as he must care for his car). You also could use the analogy to show that an excess of glucose (hyperglycemia), just like an excess of gasoline, will spill over and can be measured, and that the body, like a car, will not run without fuel (hypoglycemia).

The next section would contain a simple illustration of the four elements that affect the blood sugar level — food, insulin, exercise, and stress. Use this as a jumping-off point to develop the patient's conceptual understanding of diabetes management and to develop his problem-solving skills regarding such questions as: Should he exercise before or after meals? Why must he eat his meals on time? What will happen if he gets the flu?

Also included in this section would be a simple chart about high and low blood sugar levels. It would outline the causes, quickness of onset, signs (including urine test results), and treatment of both conditions. In discussing this section, emphasize prevention. To make sure the patient thoroughly understands the causes and effects of high and low blood sugar levels, refer back to the problem-solving skills you taught in the last section. If the patient is taking insulin or oral agents, make certain he knows what an insulin reaction is and how to treat it.

Two pictures of how to cut toenails and how not to cut them would come next, reinforcing your audiovisual or photographic program.

Finally, the pamphlet could contain pictures and information on the types of identification bracelets and necklaces available. Suggest that the patient select a bracelet, since it is more visible than a necklace. Also suggest that he choose an identification with the words "I am a diabetic" printed on it. It is more apt to catch attention in a crisis than a wallet card.

• *Insulin and You.* This handout, directed solely at the insulin-dependent patient, would briefly summarize all the insulin-related instructions from the educational program: types and concentrations of insulin, drawing up insulin, giving an injection, urine testing for insulin-dependent patients, adjusting insulin dosages, and self-care during sick days (vital information that is often neglected). It also could include a site rotation chart and a chart for recording urine tests.

If your patient is non-insulin dependent, you should give him a sheet explaining urine testing and a chart for recording results.

REPORT OF URINE TESTS

Patient's full name _____

Type of test(s) _____ Time(s) _____

Date 19____ Month, day	Urine tests				Medication	Remarks
	Breakfast	Noon meal	Supper	At bedtime		Other comments

Both *Diabetes and You* and *Insulin and You* need not be elaborate pamphlets. You could make them by simply Xeroxing or mimeographing typed pages and stapling them together.

In addition to the patient-education material, you should have a Diabetes Assessment Sheet for your own use. This sheet would contain all possible topics that you might discuss with the patient and his family. One column should be headed "Assessment," where you could record the results of your initial interview with the patient and the points you'll need to cover with other nursing personnel. Initial and date the second column, "Instruction," when you've covered the education program with the patient. Check the next three columns, "Patient Comprehends," "Patient Demonstrates," and "Family Instructed," when appropriate. Finally, leave a blank space in your assessment sheet where you can record notes. An assessment sheet will keep all of the staff informed about the teaching plan and can be used for a patient audit. Use it while the patient is in the hospital and again after he is discharged; that way, you'll ensure continuity of care and you can judge how much of his inpatient instructions he has retained.

Throughout your program, remember that teaching aids are by no means a substitute for your individualized instructions. Rather, you should use them to complement your instructions. Remember that your primary goal is to work with the patient to help him establish his own goals for self-care, using your instructional program as background. Only if he understands and helps establish his daily regimen can you expect wise and willing self-care from him.

Concentrations of insulin

1. There are three concentrations of insulin: U-40, U-80, and U-100. The concentration refers to the number of units of insulin protein in 1 ml solution.

2. U-40 insulin contains 40 units of insulin in a syringe. The bottle has a red label, cap, and letters. The syringe also has red markings. Use only a U-40 syringe with U-40 insulin.

3. U-80 insulin contains 80 units of insulin in a syringe. The bottle has a green label, cap, and letters. The syringe also has green markings. Use only a U-80 syringe with U-80 insulin.

4. U-100 insulin contains 100 units of insulin in a syringe. The bottle has black letters and an orange cap. The syringe also has black and orange markings. Use only a U-100 syringe with U-100 insulin.

5. Always match the syringe with the concentration of insulin. For example, use only a U-100 syringe with U-100 insulin. If you don't, you'll take the wrong amount of insulin.

Types of insulin

1. There are different types of insulin, such as Regular, NPH or Lente. The insulins act over different periods of time.

2. The most common short-acting insulin is Regular insulin. Regular insulin's onset, or when it begins to work, is 20-30 minutes after injection. Its peak, or when it works best, is 3 to 5 hours. Its duration, or when it is all gone, is 5 to 8 hours.

If you use only Regular insulin, you will have to take an injection before each meal.

3. The most common intermediate-acting insulins are NPH and Lente.

NPH insulin's onset is 1 to 1½ hours after injection. Its peak is 8 to 12 hours. Its duration is 24 to 28 hours.

Lente insulin's onset is 1 to 1½ hours after injection. Its peak is 8

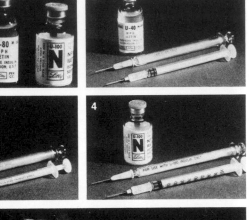

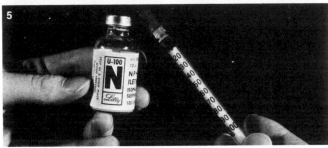

Photos by Robert Zelm

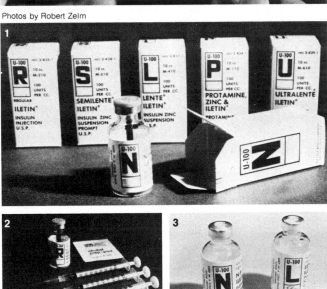

to 12 hours. Its duration is 24 to 28 hours.

With either type, you would most likely have an insulin reaction in the late afternoon, when the insulin is peaking. Eat an afternoon snack and carry candy to treat a reaction. Also eat a snack every night to prevent insulin reactions while you sleep.

4. If you use NPH or Lente insulin, you may take only one injection a day.

5. You may need to take two types of insulin, a short-acting and an intermediate-acting insulin. For example, you may be taking Regular plus NPH insulin. The activity would look like this. The Regular insulin is used because it peaks at noon, and the NPH does not peak until the late afternoon.

Always use the correct type of insulin and know when it acts. Check your insulin before you fill your syringe.

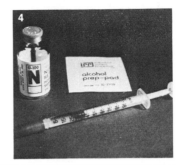

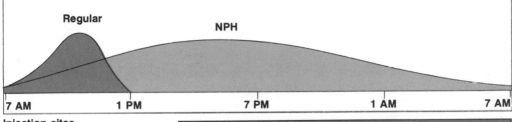

Injection sites

Insulin injections may be given in areas that have a thick layer of fat and are free from large blood vessels and nerves. You may safely use your arms, abdomen, thighs, and buttocks.

Do not use the same spot for injection more than once every 2 months. It is important to "rotate sites," or alternate areas to prevent changes in the fatty tissue that can interfere with the absorption of insulin.

1. Use this chart to help you remember where to give your injection, as well as to record that you gave it.

2. Start with spot A1 for your injection. The next day, use spot A2. Continue using spots A3 to A7 in the same manner.

Next, use the spots on your right abdomen, B1 through B7, as before. In the same manner, use your thighs and buttocks.

You may need to add or subtract spots, depending upon the amount of fat that you have. For example, if you have a large stomach, you can add more spots there.

1	INJECTION RECORD		1	2	3	4	5	6	7
SITE									
Right arm	A								
Right abdomen	B								
Right thigh	C								
Left thigh	D								
Left abdomen	E								
Left arm	F								
Left buttock	G								
Right buttock	H								

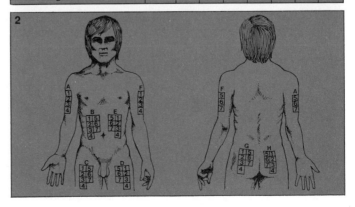

3. Measure the area on your arm with your hand. Place your hand on your shoulder and draw an imaginary line beneath your hand.
4. Place your hand above your elbow and draw an imaginary line above your hand.
5. Use the middle and outer area of your arm between these lines.
6. Measure the area on your thigh with your hand. Place your hand on your knee and draw a line

above it. Place your hand on your hip bone and draw a line below it.
7. Use the middle and outer area of your thigh between these lines.
8. Measure the area on your abdomen with your hand. Place your hands on your lower ribs and draw a line.
9. Place your hands on your hip bones and draw a line.
10. Use the area between these two lines, as far around as you can

pinch up fat. Do not use a one-inch area around your navel, nor the belt line.
11. You may also use your buttocks or upper shoulders if you have enough fat to pinch up.

If you are using an area for the first time, the insulin may be absorbed better. You could have an insulin reaction. Remember to carry candy to treat an insulin reaction.

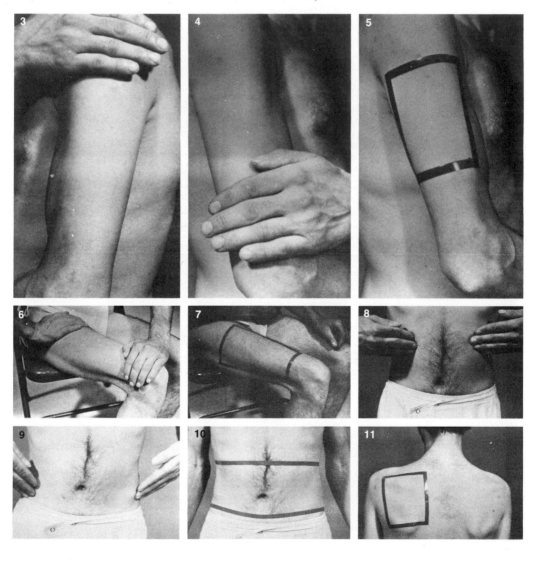

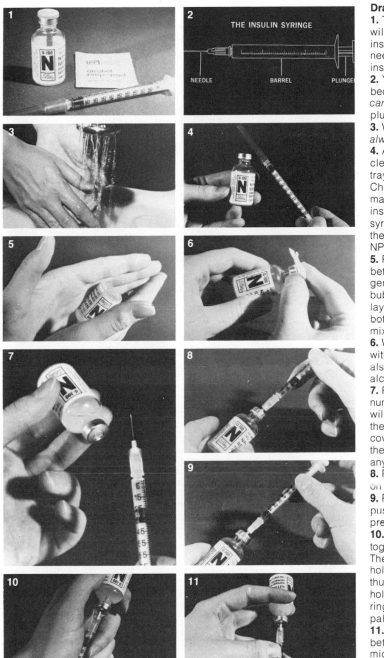

Drawing up insulin

1. This is the equipment that you will need to draw up insulin, or put insulin into the syringe. You will need a sterile syringe and needle, insulin, and an alcohol swab.

2. You cannot touch the needle because it will enter the body. You *can* touch the barrel and the plunger of the syringe.

3. Wash your hands. This is *always* the first step.

4. Assemble your equipment in a clean area. You may use a pan or tray to hold your equipment. Check that the insulin and syringe match. If you are using U-100 insulin, you must use a U-100 syringe. Also, check that you have the correct type of insulin, such as NPH or Lente.

5. Roll the bottle of insulin between your hands to mix it. Mix gently to prevent large air bubbles in the insulin. A white layer may form at the bottom of the bottle of insulin; this must be mixed.

6. Wipe off the top of the bottle with an alcohol swab. You may also use a cotton ball and rubbing alcohol.

7. Pull the plunger out to the same number of units of insulin that you will take out. This will pull air into the syringe. Take off the needle cover. The needle cover protects the needle from touching anything.

8. Put the needle into the rubber on top of the bottle of insulin.

9. Push the plunger in. This will push air into the bottle and prevent a vacuum.

10. Hold the bottle and syringe together. Turn them upside down. The bottle is now on top. You may hold the bottle between your thumb and forefinger, while holding the syringe between your ring and little fingers, against the palm of your hand.

11. You may also hold the bottle between your forefinger and middle finger, while holding the syringe between your thumb and little finger.

12. Pull back on the plunger to the correct number of units of insulin.

13. Check for air bubbles. (Air is clear. NPH and Lente insulin are cloudy; Regular insulin is clear.) Air bubbles will not harm you, *but* they may prevent you from taking the correct amount of insulin.

14. Remove air bubbles by pulling out the plunger further. Push the plunger back to the correct number of units of insulin. This will push the air back into the bottle. (You may not be able to remove all of the tiny air bubbles.)

15. You also may flick the barrel of the syringe sharply with your middle finger.

16. Or, you may push the plunger back in. This will push the air and insulin back into the bottle. Pull the plunger out again to the correct number of units of insulin.

Check that the syringe contains the correct amount of insulin and there are no air bubbles. If there are no bubbles, and the correct amount of insulin is in the syringe, take the needle out of the bottle.

17. Put the cover back on the needle. This will protect the needle until you are ready to give yourself the injection.

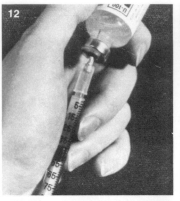

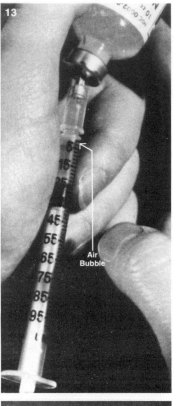

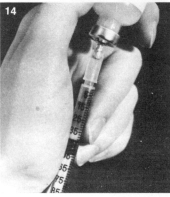

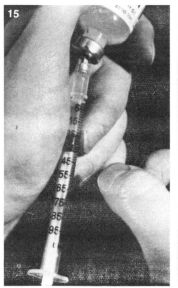

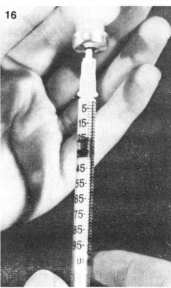

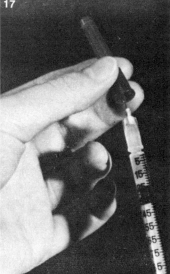

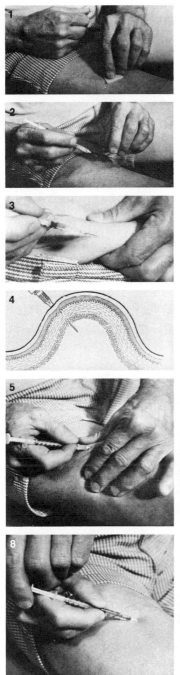

Injecting insulin

Use your injection chart to find the spot where you will give yourself the injection or shot of insulin.

1. Wipe off the spot with an alcohol swab. You may also use a cotton ball and alcohol to clean the spot.

2. Take the cover off the needle and put it aside temporarily. Hold the syringe like a pencil.

3. Grasp the spot where you will give the injection between the thumb and fingers of your free hand. Pinch up firmly!

To pinch up the spot on your arm, press the back of your upper arm against a chair back or corner of a wall. "Roll" your arm down.

4. Pinching up the spot will pull the fat away from the muscle. The injection will be into the fat.

5. Put the needle into the spot with a jab, like throwing a dart. Do not *push* the needle in. If your syringe has a long needle, insert it at a 45° angle, all the way to the end of the needle.

6. You may also spread the skin between your fingers and insert the needle straight up and down.

Use this technique if you have more fat. If you're using a syringe with a short (½") needle, insert it straight into the skin.

7. Let go of the spot and use that hand to pull back on the plunger about two units. Check for blood near the needle. If there is no blood, push the plunger in.

8. If you see blood, the needle is in a small blood vessel. Pull the needle out and put it into another spot, as before. Check for blood again. If there is no blood, push the plunger in. If you see blood, pull the needle out and throw away the syringe. Draw up a new syringe of insulin and use this for your injection.

9. Place the alcohol swab over the needle, after you have pushed the plunger in. Pull the needle out quickly and press the swab over the spot for two seconds. Put the cover on the needle.

10. Break the needle off by quickly snapping the syringe and needle together, like breaking a stick. Throw away the syringe and needle. Write on the chart where you took the shot.

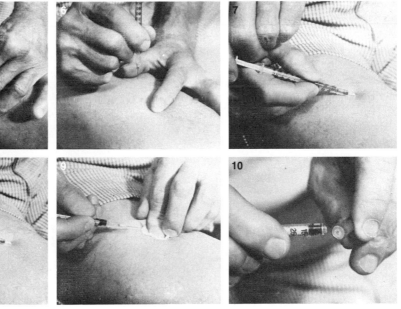

Daily foot care

As you grow older, the circulation to your feet decreases. This is especially true for the diabetic. With decreased circulation, your body can't heal injuries to your feet. An ingrown toenail or blister can lead to an infection. The nerves in your feet that tell you if something is too hot or too cold may also be affected. You may burn yourself and not know it. So, taking care of your feet every day is important to prevent foot problems.

Always take care of your feet every day at the same time. This will help you to remember to do it. Choose the time of day that is best for you.

1. This is the equipment that you will need: a basin, washcloth and towel, mild soap, shoes, and socks. You may also use a bathtub or shower.

2. Wash your feet in warm water. Always check the temperature of the water with your hand or elbow before putting your feet in. This will prevent burns from water that is too hot.

3. Soak your feet for 5 to 10 minutes.

4. Soap up the washcloth. Use it to wash your whole foot, especially between your toes and around your toenails.

5. Dry your feet gently by blotting them with a towel. Be sure to dry between your toes.

6. If your have dry skin, it may look like this.

7. Apply oil or lotion to your feet immediately after washing and drying. This will prevent the water from evaporating and drying your skin. The lotion will keep your skin soft.

If you have sweaty feet, use a mild foot powder. Put it between your toes, in your socks, and in your shoes.

8. Inspect your feet every day for injuries. This is just as important as washing your feet. With decreased feeling in your feet, you may not feel an injury. Injuries include pressure from shoes that are too tight, a cut on a toe, or stepping on a tack. Look between your toes, around the toenails, and at every part of your foot for cracks, blisters, corns, calluses, and red and swollen areas. If you find an injury, wash the area with warm, soapy water. You may use a mild antiseptic, such as Bactine, but don't use harsh antiseptics, such as iodine. Do not use your injured foot. Elevate it as often as possible. This will help the circulation to heal the injury.

If an injury becomes infected, it will be red, swollen, painful, and hot, and may ooze pus. Call your doctor immediately if an injury doesn't heal or becomes infected.

9. You can also injure yourself by cutting corns and calluses or using a liquid corn remover. You may cut too deeply or the corn remover may burn too deeply. If you have corns and calluses, rub them with a towel after washing your feet. This will avoid injury. To get rid of corns or calluses, consult a podiatrist.

10. Wear clean socks every day. Cotton or wool socks absorb perspiration best. Socks should be smooth and have loose tops. A tight top could cut off circulation to your feet. You may wear either white socks or colored socks, as long as the dye is colorfast.

Always wear leather shoes. (Leather shoes allow your feet to "breathe"; plastic shoes cause your feet to perspire and can lead to fungal infections, blisters, and rashes.) Make sure your shoes have ties or buckles with a low heel and are properly fitted. Buy them at the end of the day, when your feet will be the largest. Break in new shoes gradually, wearing them one-half hour a day. If possible, have several pairs and wear a different pair each day.

Before putting on your shoes, check inside them for objects, rough spots, or torn linings, which could injure your feet.

Never go barefoot or wear shoes without socks. Socks and shoes protect your feet from injury.

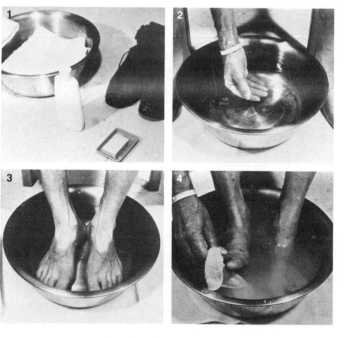

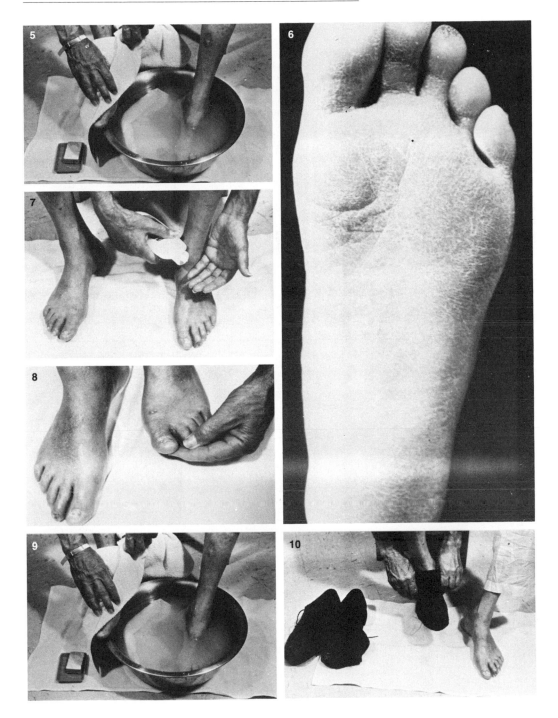

Cutting toenails

Many people have difficulty cutting their toenails. Their toenails may be thick, tough, or misshapen. Or they may have difficulty seeing or reaching their toenails to cut them safely. If you have any of these difficulties, ask a member of your family, a nurse, or a doctor to cut your toenails for you, or see a podiatrist.

1. This is the equipment that you will need: a basin, towel, emery board, and nippers, scissors, or a clipper with a straight edge.

2. Soak your feet in warm water. Check the temperature of the water with your hand or elbow before putting your feet in. Soak your feet for at least 15 minutes. This will soften your toenails. Dry your feet gently by blotting them with a towel. (You may want to cut your toenails during your daily foot care, after washing and drying your feet.)

3. When cutting, use only the end of the nipper or scissor's blade. This will prevent splitting of the nail.

4. Take short "bites" across the nail. Start at the corner, cutting the nail straight across, even with the end of the toe.

5. If you cut into the corners, you may cut a hook that will dig into the toe as the nail grows. Likewise, if you cut the nail too short, it will also dig into the toe as the nail grows.

6. File any ragged edge with an emery board. This will prevent the toenails from digging into adjacent toes and from tearing the stockings. If you can't cut your toenails because they are thick and tough, file your toenails with an emery board every day after washing and drying your feet. This will prevent the need to cut your toenails.

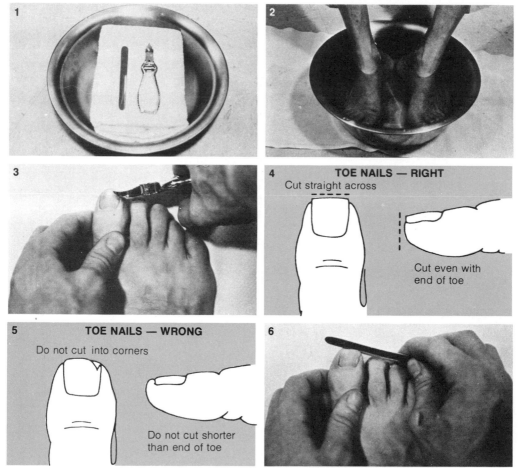

Urine testing

Tapes such as Tes-Tape, Clinistix, and Diastix test the urine for glucose. Tapes such as Keto-Diastix test the urine for ketones as well as glucose. You may find ketones in urine if you are losing weight, are sick, or have very high blood glucose.

1. The color chart for a urine test is on the bottle. For a Diastix or Keto-Diastix glucose test, the blue color indicates no glucose (negative) and the dark brown color indicates a large amount of glucose (4+). Clinistix and Tes-Tape have similar color charts. For a Keto-Diastix ketone test, the buff color indicates no ketones (negative) and the dark purple color indicates a large amount of ketones.

2. All urine test strips are affected by humidity and sunlight. Always keep the cap tight and store the bottle out of direct sunlight.

3. Remove a strip from the bottle; tightly close the cap. (With Tes-Tape, tear off about 1½ inches.)

4. To test urine, hold the strip at the end that doesn't have the color blocks, making sure that the printing is facing you. Do not touch the color blocks.

5. Dip the strip into the container of urine for at least 2 seconds. The color blocks must be thoroughly wet. Take the strip out of the urine. Tap it against the side of the container to remove excess urine. Begin timing.

6. When using Keto-Diastix, compare the buff color with the ketone color chart *exactly 15 seconds* after removing the strip from the urine. Read the color blocks *only* from the side with the printing. (The glue on the back of the blocks interferes with the test.)

7. When using Diastix or Keto-Stix, compare the blue color block to the glucose color chart *exactly 30 seconds* after removing the strip from the urine. The color may change after 30 seconds, so record the color *only* at 30 seconds. When using Clinistix, compare colors *exactly 10 seconds* after removing the strip. When using Tes-Tape, compare the darkest part of the tape *exactly 1 minute* after removing.

8. Your doctor may have you test urine with a 2- or 5-drop tablet test, such as Clinitest. To do so, collect urine in a clean receptacle. Using the dropper, place 2 or 5 drops of urine in a test tube. Rinse the dropper and add 10 drops of water. Drop a tablet into the test tube. Watch *during boiling and for 15 seconds after boiling stops*. Then shake the tube gently and match the color chart.

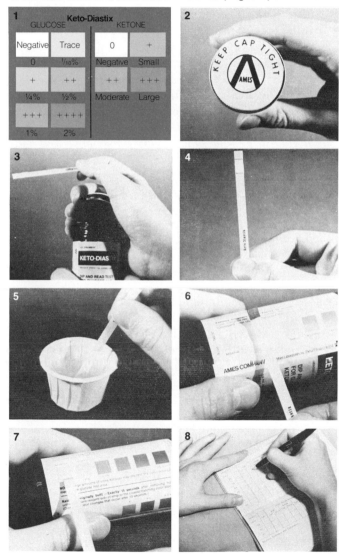

Urine testing for insulin-dependent patients
If you are controlling your diabetes by diet and insulin, test your urine for *glucose* four times a day. Test it before breakfast, lunch, dinner, and bedtime.

The urine you test should be "double-voided" — that is, urine that has just been filtered by the kidneys.
• Urinate (this will rid your body of all urine)
• Drink a glass of water
• Urinate again 30 minutes later into a clean container
• Test the second urine.

Always write down your urine test results. Use a record of them to adjust your insulin, diet, and exercise. Bring this record when you see the doctor. Your urine tests should read negative to 1+. If all of your urine tests are negative, you don't know the level of glucose in your blood. It may be too low, so you might have insulin reactions.

Test your urine four times a day for glucose and ketones when:
• Your urine is 3+ or 4+
• You are having signs of high blood sugar, such as excessive thirst, urination, or fatigue
• You are under physical stress, such as a cold or the flu.
  Call your doctor when:
• Your urine stays at 4+ for 2 days
• Your urine contains ketones.

Urine testing for non-insulin dependent patients
If you are controlling your diabetes by diet, or by diet and medication, test your urine for *glucose* once a day. Test it about 2 hours after the largest meal of the day. This will test the urine that has been made *after* eating. This is also the time you are most likely to have glucose in the urine.

Write down your urine test results. Bring a record of them when you see the doctor.

Your urine should always test negative.

Test your urine four times a day for glucose when:
• Your urine is 3+ or 4+
• You are having signs of high blood sugar, such as excessive thirst, urination, or fatigue
• You are under physical stress, such as a cold or the flu.
  Call your doctor if:
• Your urine tests are 4+ for 2 days.

7

REFINING URINE TEST TACTICS

BY DELORES SCHUMANN, RN, MS

LIKE MANY nurses, you may find urine tests for glucosuria a snap to perform. Yet studies suggest that many nurses neglect to pass along the fine points of urine testing to their patients.

The preceding chapter graphically showed how a patient should conduct a urine test. But to help ensure that he gets accurate test results, you also should explain these "refinements" of urine testing.

Glucosuria, the presence of glucose in the urine, depends on two things: the plasma glucose level, and the renal threshold (the point of blood glucose concentration at which the kidney excretes glucose). Normally, glucosuria doesn't occur until the renal threshold exceeds 180 mg/100 ml. But you should be aware of the exceptions. Diabetics (particularly the younger and the well-controlled) and elderly persons, who have elevated renal thresholds, could have negative urine tests even though their plasma glucose is high. Conversely, an occasional diabetic patient will have a low renal threshold. He'll test positive to glucosuria even though his plasma glucose is not elevated.

Glucosuria tests consist of two main types: reducing and enzyme. Reducing tests (e.g., Clinitest, Benedict's test) react with sugars other than glucose. That is, they develop a positive reaction if galactose, lactose, maltose, or pentose is present in

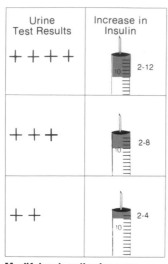

Urine Test Results	Increase in Insulin
+ + + +	2-12
+ + +	2-8
+ +	2-4

Modifying insulin dosages
The above chart is a handy reference for how to apply urine test results to insulin dose modification. For example, if your patient's test result is 4+, he should increase his insulin by 2 to 12 units; if it is 3+, he should increase it 2 to 8 units; and if it is 2+, he should increase it 2 to 4 units.

the urine. Enzyme tests (e.g., Tes-Tape, Clinistix, Diastix) respond specifically to glucose by producing a color change on a paper strip or stick.

You should be aware of the basic differences between these tests to choose the appropriate one for your diabetic patient. For example, nursing mothers and women in their third trimester of pregnancy have lactose in their urine, so they should use an enzyme test, such as Tes-Tape, because it checks only for glucose.

With the enzyme tests, the patient compares the color change on the test strip to a reference color chart supplied by the manufacturer. He should use only charts with bright colors; faded color charts won't allow him to distinguish adequately between color sequences.

The color charts distributed by the various manufacturers are not interchangeable. For example, the color sequences on the charts for Clinitest and Tes-Tape are just the reverse of each other — orange indicates a negative response to Tes-Tape, but it suggests a 2% concentration of glucose for Clinitest.

Glucosuria test results are often recorded with a plus symbol (+) but the number of pluses for various percentages of glucose is not standarized (see Table 1). For example, a 3-plus result for Tes-Tape indicates ½% glucose, but a 3-plus for Clinitest indicates 1% glucose. The Clinistix test does not use the plus system at all, but rather a system of color gradation from light to dark. (Thus, to ensure accuracy in the hospital, you should record urine test results by percent of glucose present rather than by pluses. And most important — be sure to specify which test was used. If you test a patient with Clinitest tablets and the evening nurse uses Tes-Tape, determining the exact amount of glucose that patient is excreting becomes impossible. And, the inconsistency in test results would cause erratic regulation of insulin dosage.)

How drugs affect glucosuria tests
Drugs containing sugar. If a diabetic begins to show glucose in his urine after he has started taking a new medication, he should check to see whether that drug contains sugar and if so, the type of sugar. Many medicinal agents contain sweeteners, flavoring agents, or fillers that have a high sugar content (see Table 2). Elixirs, suspensions, and syrups (e.g., cough syrups,

TABLE 1 — DIFFERENCES AMONG URINE TESTS FOR GLUCOSE

Glucose Concentration

TEST	0%	1/10%	1/4%	1/2%	3/4%	1%	2%	2%
Benedict's	Neg	Trace	+		++		+++	++++
Diastix	Neg	Trace	+	++		+++	++++	
Tes-Tape	Neg	+	++	+++			++++	
Clinitest	Neg		Trace	+	++	+++	++++	
Clinistix	light		medium		dark			

TABLE 2 — AMOUNT AND TYPE OF SUGAR IN SELECTED MEDICATIONS

MEDICATION AND DOSAGE FORM	GM/5 ML SUGAR	TYPE OF SUGAR
Actified (syrup)	3.5	Sucrose
Keflex (supension)	3.0	Sucrose
Penbritin — 250 mg bottle (suspension)	2.195	Sucrose
Quibron (elixir)	2.25	Sucrose
Robitussin (syrup)	2.8	Glucose/sucrose
V-Cillin K 250 (solution)	3.0	Sucrose
Vi-Daylin (liquid)	4.85	Glucose/sucrose
Zymatinic (drops)	2.994	Sucrose

antibiotic suspensions) often have sugar as part of their base. If a diabetic takes these drugs, he may ingest a substantially higher amount of carbohydrate than his prescribed diet allows. The added glucose intake will, of course, show up in his glucosuria test.

Ascorbic acid and aspirin. Diabetics who consume large quantities of ascorbic acid (vitamin C) or aspirin should know that they may have positive urine tests even though glucose is not present. Since these drugs are used so widely, and with relative safety, they're not often thought of as problem sources.

Large quantities of vitamin C can creep into a diet in subtle ways. Because this vitamin is popularly credited with such a

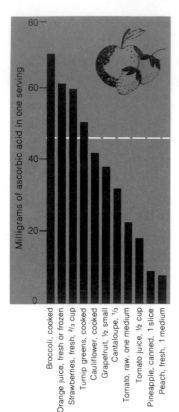

Watch out for Vitamin C!
In the above chart the dashed line represents the recommended daily allowance of ascorbic acid. A high amount of Vitamin C in the diet can give falsely negative urine tests. With Clinistix, if there is 0.1% glucose in the patient's urine, between 10-20 mg/100 ml of Vitamin C can give a falsely negative reading. Warn your patient to keep an eye on how much Vitamin C he eats. If your patient questions the accuracy of his urine test and has been consuming large quantities of Vitamin C, suggest that he retest with Diastix or Clinitest, which is less sensitive to Vitamin C.

wide range of therapeutic properties, even a diabetic who's aware of the restrictions imposed on his diet might take it. For instance, he might take multiple vitamin or iron preparations, which contain varying amounts of vitamin C, without his physician's recommendation or knowledge. Or he could be getting large amounts of this vitamin from fruits, fruit drinks, or foods that have been fortified with vitamin C as the food preservative and antioxidant. Still another source is intravenous tetracycline preparations, which are buffered with ascorbic acid.

Aspirin produces false positive glucosuria test results through the metabolite, gentisic acid. Since only about 1% to 8% of aspirin is converted to gentisic acid, a casual dose wouldn't affect test results. But 2.4 grams, or seven tablets, of aspirin per day *could* produce enough gentisic acid in the urine to affect the measurement of glucosuria. This means that patients who take aspirin regularly — for arthritis, for instance — can have enough gentisic acid to affect urine tests.

Other affecting drugs. A patient should always be sure to check the manufacturer's insert packaged with the test materials to see which specific drugs are known to affect test results. Clinitest, for example, will indicate false positive results if he is taking sufficient concentrations of: nalidixic acid (NegGram), cephalosporin antibiotics (Keflin, Keflex, and Loridine), probenecid (Benemid), or vitamin C (ascorbic acid). Drugs known to alter results with Tes-Tape are: dipyrone (Narone and Pyrilgin), meralluride (Mercuhydrin), levodopa (Dopar, Larodopa, and Bendopa), methyldopa (Aldomet), aspirin, and ascorbic acid. If a patient is taking any of these medications, he should ask his doctor to switch him to a urine test that isn't affected by the medication.

Second-voided specimens

An insulin-dependent diabetic must use the second-voided specimen for his urine test. This means that he empties his bladder of all urine, drinks some water, and voids again about a half hour later, providing the specimen for the glucosuria test. This specimen should reflect the level of plasma glucose between the two voiding periods as urine was collecting in the bladder.

If second-voided specimens are persistently positive for glucosuria but the plasma glucose levels are low, the patient may not have completely emptied his bladder. This could be caused by damage to the nerves supplying the bladder (neurogenic bladder) or by an enlarged prostate. Whatever the cause, the glucose content of the residual urine will be reflected in all of the patient's specimens.

The practice of encouraging patients to drink water between the first and second voidings also may contribute to misleading glucosuria test results. A recent study, for example, disclosed that diluted urine was a significant factor in overestimating glucosuria. In all four tests used — Clinitest, Tes-Tape, Clinistix, and Diastix — glucose content was overestimated in second-voided specimens; Clinitest overestimated more than the others. The reason why this occurred has not been explored. Nevertheless, you should keep abreast of research findings in this area to increase your competence in teaching urine testing for glucosuria.

Misuse of test materials

A patient should never use test materials that have a past expiration date, are discolored, or have been exposed to moisture. Moisture, perhaps more than anything else, causes deterioration of test materials.

His own handling of test materials is important. He shouldn't leave Tes-Tape strips lying on utility room sinks, bathroom shelves, or near water faucets. Nor should he leave tablet and enzyme strip bottles uncovered from one test time to the next. Since most test materials come in jars with screw-top lids and with a desiccant to minimize moisturizing effects, he must be sure to use them. He can protect the Tes-Tape dispenser by keeping it in a small jar with a screw-top lid between uses.

Following directions. The patient must always read the directions accompanying the test materials and follow them precisely. For example, he must hold a Tes-Tape strip in the air during the reaction. If he lays it on a piece of paper, small amounts of glucose from the paper could affect the results. And he should *never* dip the strip in urine and then blot the excess by brushing it against a paper towel.

Be sure he knows to wait the specified length of time before he reads the test results. This is especially important with Clinitest. He must watch the Clinitest reaction during its entire process and for 15 seconds after it stops boiling inside the tube.

Reliability tests

A patient can detect deterioration in some test materials by a change in the color of the agent (e.g., Tes-Tape becomes brown, while Clinitest tablets change from a robin's egg blue to a dark, speckled color and eventually to black). But a test agent can deteriorate without changing color. So if he has any reason to suspect its reliability, he should check it in a glucose solution. The test material should give a reading of 2% or more glucose. A "suitable glucose solution" might be a freshly opened bottle or can of cola that contains sugar. Make sure the patient knows not to use dietetic colas, though, as their glucose content differs from that of regular colas. Table sugar is not suitable for this purpose, either, since it is sucrose, not glucose.

DOSAGE ADJUSTMENTS FOR SOME PATTERNS OF GLUCOSURIA

UNITS OF INSULIN	PATTERNS OF GLUCOSURIA				DOSAGE ADJUSTMENT
	7 a.m.	11 a.m.	4 p.m.	9 p.m.	
1. 20 NPH	trace	4+	0	0	16 NPH + 4 Regular, a.m.
2. 16 NPH + 4 Regular	trace	4+	1+	trace	16 NPH + 6-8 Regular, a.m.
3. 16 NPH + 8 Regular	1	trace	3+	4+	20-22 NPH + 8 Regular, a.m.
4. 16 NPH + 8 Regular	0	0	trace	4+	20-22 NPH +4-6 Regular, a.m.
5. 16 NPH + 4 Regular	0	0	0	0	14 NPH + 4 Regular
6. 18 NPH + 4 Regular	4	3	1	1	(a) Substitute Lente insulin for NPH in a.m. (b) Retain present a.m. dose and give 4 to 6 units of NPH insulin before supper. (c) Add a long-acting phenformin (50 mg.) at supper time. (d) Substitute an equal amount of long-acting insulin for the NPH, and increase the Regular insulin 4 units.
7. 20 NPH + 4 Regular	4+	4+	4+	4+	*If no acute complications:* 24 NPH + 8 Regular, a.m.+ 4-6 NPH before supper. *If acute complications present:* 12 Regular at 7 a.m., 1 p.m., 7 p.m., 1 a.m.

If the color changes rapidly from green to tan to orange to a dark greenish-brown (this is known as pass-through color change), the urine has a glucose concentration greater than 2%. The patient shouldn't try to compare these results to the regular color chart.

If he is using the 2-drop method be sure that he has the special color chart for it. Remind him that these charts are not available at local drug stores; they must be obtained from the manufacturer. And be sure to warn your patient that whenever he buys a new bottle of Clinitest tablets he should discard the five-drop color chart in the package and use only the special two-drop color chart.

Testing for ketone bodies
There are three types of ketone bodies — 2% acetone, 20% acetoacetate, and 88% betahydroxybutyrate — and small

amounts of these may normally be present in the urine. Like glucose, however, ketones are usually excreted into the urine only after they reach a threshold level in the blood.

Ketonuria occurs not only in diabetics but also in nondiabetic persons as a result of reducing diets or eating a high-fat, high-protein but low-carbohydrate diet. Fasting, pregnancy, lactation, and severe infections accompanied by vomiting and diarrhea can cause positive results in ketone tests. On the other hand, severe dehydration or advanced kidney disease may produce a high level of ketone bodies in the blood but the amount excreted into the urine will not reflect the excessive level.

To test for ketone bodies, a freshly voided urine specimen is required. This is because urine that stands at room temperature stimulates bacterial growth, causing changes in the amount of ketones.

A single test does not check all three ketone bodies. For instance, the "quick" testing materials for diabetics check for acetoacetate alone or the combination of acetoacetate and acetone. Thus, if the excreted ketone bodies are largely beta-hydroxybutyrate, the test will not reflect the extent of the ketogenesis (the production of ketone bodies).

Although ketonuria is a warning signal for the diabetic that control of his condition is wavering, it doesn't necessarily indicate impending ketoacidosis. For safety's sake, then, when should the diabetic check for ketones? If he shows negative or trace amounts of glucose in his urine, he needn't check routinely for ketone bodies. But he should check for ketones if he begins to show a concentration of ¾% or more — or according to many specialists, a 2% (4+) concentration more than two times in succession, or during illness. He should continue this testing every 3 to 4 hours until the ketone bodies are no longer present.

Routine testing for ketone bodies should be done by diabetics who (1) have not attained good control or who are "brittle"; (2) experience loss of weight or stress, due to vigorous exercise, exposure to cold, digestive disturbances, surgery or illness; or (3) are newly diagnosed and whose health status needs to be assessed. Also, you should encourage the insulin-dependent diabetic to check for ketones occasionally so he doesn't forget the techniques of the testing method.

The same precautions that apply to glucosuria tests also apply to ketone test materials. That is, the patient shouldn't expose them to moisture, direct sunlight, or heat. If strips or tablets become discolored, he should destroy them, since this indicates loss of sensitivity. He also should check to see what drugs can affect results — e.g., aspirin or a Bromsulphalein test can produce false positive results with Ketostix. And again, he should always follow directions explicitly.

Selecting the right test
When you select a testing method for your patient's self-use, remember that no test will fit all situations. First, assess the patient's health history as well as his ability to manage his condition. Then select a method that he can perform correctly. Finally, check the medications that can affect this test and find out whether your patient is taking any of them. If so, you'll need to either select a different test or warn the patient not to continue taking the medications.

By putting these tips into practice, you'll be aiding your patients to achieve more accurate urine testing results.

8

EXPLAINING AXIOMS FOR SICK DAYS

BY JUDITH C. PETROKAS, RN

MILD, SEEMINGLY UNIMPORTANT illnesses such as diarrhea or gastrointestinal upset pose no serious threat to normally healthy people. But they can pose serious problems to diabetics, particularly insulin-dependent diabetics. Because these illnesses affect food intake, which affects insulin needs.

Consider, for example, what happened to Mrs. Armstrong, a newly diagnosed diabetic, who came down with the flu. Since she couldn't tolerate any food and feared having an insulin reaction, she decided to omit her insulin. Feeling too ill to test her urine, she failed to notice her elevated blood sugar and the appearance of ketones in her urine.

After 8 hours without food or insulin, Mrs. Armstrong became short of breath, very tired, excessively thirsty, and experienced more nausea, vomiting, and frequent urination. In fact, she felt so ill that she asked her neighbor, Mrs. Ryan, to take her to the hospital. The outcome: She was admitted with diabetic ketoacidosis.

All this could have been prevented if Mrs. Armstrong had followed a few simple guidelines on how to take care of herself during a sudden, short-term illness. But her experience wasn't unique — many insulin-dependent diabetics make the same mistake of not eating and not taking insulin when they become ill. And they end up being hospitalized. An important aspect of

Sick-day CHO
On the opposite page you will find some of the recommended foods your patient can eat when sick to maintain adequate nutrition and balance his insulin. Ginger ale, fruit juices, skim milk, cream soups, egg nog, popsicles, sherbet, ice cream, and jello are easily digested and gentle on the stomach.

working with all diabetics, therefore, is to teach them how to cope with short-term illness without sacrificing control of their diabetes.

Defining a short-term illness
The first step is to help patients distinguish between short-term and long-term illnesses. For the diabetic, a short-term illness is one in which the acute phase doesn't persist longer than 72 hours (e.g., influenza, cold, diarrhea). Or, if it does persist, the patient can tolerate most of the meat exchanges of his pre-scribed diet, plus all of the fruit, vegetable, and bread ex-changes. A long-term illness is one that persists longer than 72 hours (e.g., complications arise, or the patient shows no im-provement after this time). A diabetic who has a long-term illness should definitely see his physician.

Following are some simple guidelines for short-term ill-nesses. Be sure to explain the importance of each one and tell your patient how he can apply common sense to it.

1. *Never omit insulin.* The insulin-dependent diabetic (like Mrs. Armstrong) may fear an insulin reaction because he's unable to take his usual amount of food. So, he may decide not to take his insulin or any food except small amounts of fluids. Therefore, you must impress upon him the fact that his body *needs* insulin, despite his decreased food intake.

Explain that his physician may instruct him to use a sliding scale for Regular or short-acting insulin when he is ill. But he must not make *any other changes* in his insulin without first consulting the physician. (If your patient is taking oral agents, he shouldn't try to adjust his dosage during an illness. Tell him to simply stop taking the medication if he can't eat; otherwise, he should take them as usual.)

Also, tell the patient if he vomits or has diarrhea, he should notify his physician at once. Since vomiting and diarrhea deplete body fluids, causing electrolyte imbalance, these con-ditions must be corrected as soon as possible.

2. *Go to bed and keep warm.* Tell the patient to have someone stay with him if at all possible. If he should have an insulin reaction, having someone there who knows what to do can probably prevent it from becoming severe.

3. *Test urine for sugar and acetone at least four times a day, using the two-drop Clinitest and Ketostix.* This rule ap-plies not only to insulin-dependent diabetics but also to those

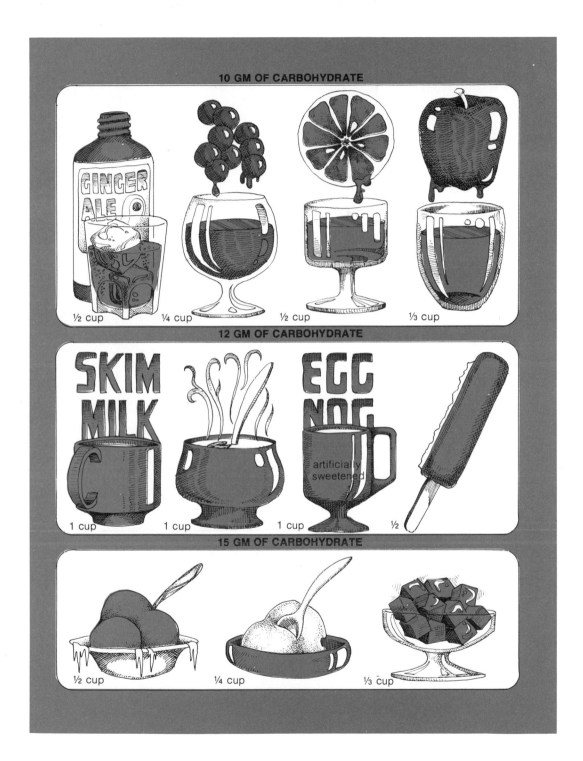

10 GM OF CARBOHYDRATE

½ cup   ¼ cup   ½ cup   ⅓ cup

12 GM OF CARBOHYDRATE

SKIM MILK   EGG NOG   artificially sweetened

1 cup   1 cup   1 cup   ½

15 GM OF CARBOHYDRATE

½ cup   ¼ cup   ⅓ cup

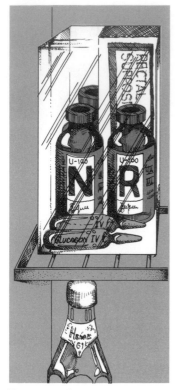

Be prepared
Tell your patient to be prepared for illness by keeping Paragoric, Maalox, Tylenol, and Milk of Magnesia in the medicine cabinet and glucagon, rectal suppositories, his usual insulin, and Regular insulin in the refrigerator.

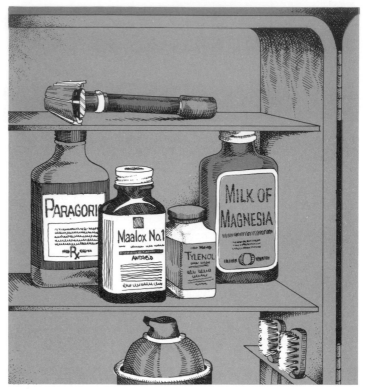

on oral agents if their doctor advises urine tests. The two-drop Clinitest is preferable to the five-drop method because it reduces the possibility of flashback. (Flashback is the bright orange color, or 5%, that appears during the boiling process. After 15 seconds, the test will show 2% or 3%. Since this happens so quickly, the patient often overlooks it, not realizing he should record the results as 5%.)

Remind your patient to use second-voided specimens for these tests and to repeat the tests every 4 to 6 hours (or every 2 to 4 hours if he's a juvenile or brittle type). Explain that the physician needs to know the results of both sugar and acetone tests to determine whether insulin should be adjusted.

4. *Take liquids every hour.* Tell the patient to keep a record of all food and fluids taken and retained and to report this information to his physician. Again, this will help the physician make necessary adjustments in type and amount of insulin.

Remind the patient that taking small amounts of liquids frequently helps replenish the fluid he loses through vomiting, diarrhea, or fever. Encourage him to take 8 ounces of liquids,

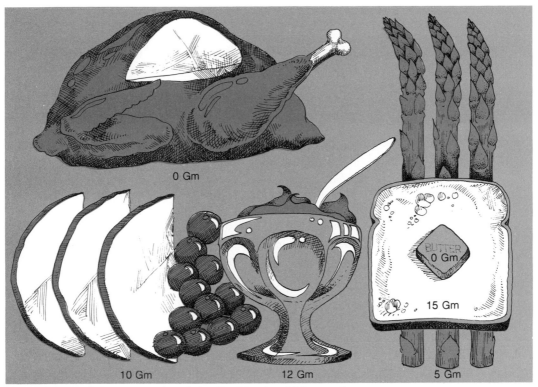

0 Gm

10 Gm

12 Gm

5 Gm

15 Gm

0 Gm

if he can. Explain that some of the liquids should be a salty broth, to replace the sodium he loses through vomiting and diarrhea. This advice applies to all diabetics, whether they're on diet, oral agents, or insulin.

5. If unable to eat the prescribed diet, replace the carbohydrate with liquid or semi-liquid foods. Remind every diabetic that carbohydrates are more easily tolerated during illness than proteins or fats, and they affect his blood sugar more rapidly. But if he can't tolerate solid food, he can replace them with liquid carbohydrates (see page 85).

6. If still unable to eat the prescribed diet after replacing four or five meals with liquid or semi-liquid carbohydrates, call the physician. Explain to your patient that his diet must be adjusted to include proteins and fats so he can maintain adequate nutrition. Teach him how to calculate replacements for his diet so his insulin dose will be balanced with food.

Applying the guidelines

Now let's see how these guidelines would have applied to Mrs. Armstrong. After taking her morning insulin, she could have

A healthy lunch for Mrs. Armstrong
When feeling well, Mrs. Armstrong has for lunch three lean meat exchanges, one fruit, one milk (yogurt), one bread, one fat, and one non-starchy vegetable exchange (about three asparagus spears), amounting to 42 grams of carbohydrate.

asked Mrs. Ryan to stay with her until her husband came home from work. Then she would have gone to bed and kept warm, taking frequent sips of tap water throughout the morning.

At lunch time, Mrs. Ryan could have helped Mrs. Armstrong test her urine. The results probably would have been negative for sugar and acetone. She could have replaced the carbohydrate in her prescribed diet with ginger ale, calculating her meal as shown on page 87.

Since ½ cup of ginger ale provides 10 Gm of carbohydrate, Mrs. Armstrong would have taken 2 cups (40 Gm). She also could have used the replacement system for her evening meal. She could have taken some bouillon at intervals to replace the sodium she had lost through vomiting, thus maintaining an electrolyte balance. By the following day, she probably would have been able to resume her prescribed diet.

Simple guidelines like these, plus thorough teaching, can help patients maintain control of their diabetes during a short-term illness. But be sure they understand that *no* guidelines can take the place of professional medical care — only a physician can provide this service. Common sense should guide your patients in deciding which course to follow.

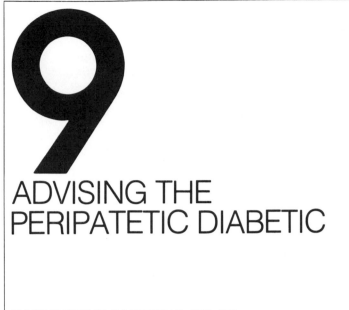

9
ADVISING THE PERIPATETIC DIABETIC

BY CATHERINE GAROFANO, RN, BS

HELPING PATIENTS MANAGE their diabetes at home involves setting up a routine. But what happens to that routine when a diabetic goes on a trip? Very simply, he takes the routine with him. Since this may pose problems, he'll need to do some preplanning and take certain precautions. Here's how you can help.

Planning ahead

First, if your patient doesn't already have some type of medical identification, urge him to get a card or tag identifying him as a diabetic and to carry it with him at all times. This identification should include his physician's name and address and the type and amount of insulin or oral agent he's currently taking.

To ensure that his trip begins without any hitches, suggest that he have a general checkup before leaving. An ordinary but undetected health problem such as an abscessed tooth could become particularly traumatic for a diabetic in unfamiliar surroundings.

If your patient needs vaccinations or immunizations, tell him to get them a few weeks earlier than usual, since any reactions could affect his diabetes' equilibrium. Of course, if this happens while he's still at home, his own physician is

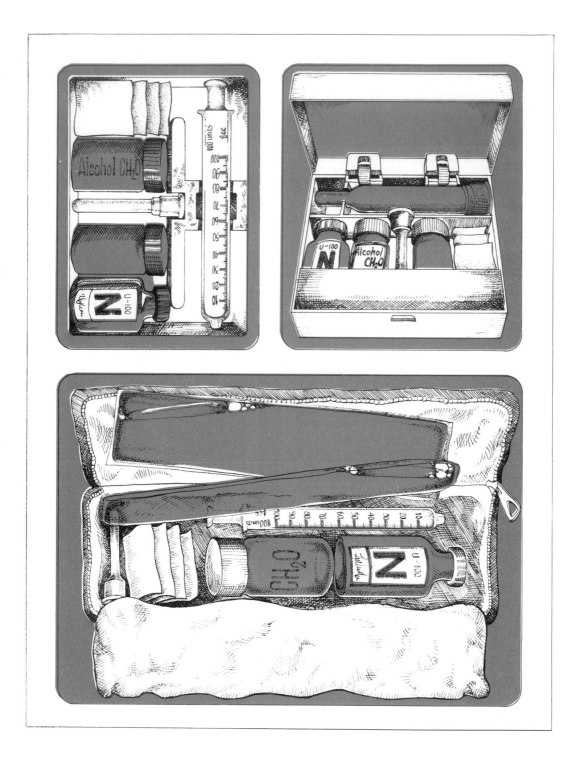

readily available to handle the situation. And having the reaction under control will ease the patient's mind when he sets out on his trip.

You might also suggest that he ask the doctor to prescribe an antidiarrheal agent that he can obtain before leaving. Again, diarrhea is disabling for people without chronic disease; think of the consequences for a diabetic!

Of course, you should advise your patient to take along enough medication to last him throughout the trip (although he can obtain foreign equivalents if necessary), as well as syringes, glucagon, and urine testing equipment. Either disposable needles and syringes or a compact kit that includes a reusable syringe, needles, cotton, and a 1-week supply of insulin is convenient for traveling.

If your patient does plan to take along standard syringes, remind him that sterilizing them could be a problem. My patients have reported that hotel kitchens aren't always prepared to give this kind of service.

Suggest that your patient get a written statement from his doctor explaining that he's a diabetic and takes insulin by injection. This, along with his medical identification, will facilitate getting syringes through customs as well as getting replacement syringes in a foreign pharmacy, if that should become necessary. (My patients, who've taken these precautions, have traveled to Europe, the Middle East, and the Caribbean without any difficulties going through customs. Diabetes is an international disease, and patients have found that most customs agents recognize medical identification tags and don't question possession of syringes and needles.)

Also, suggest that your patient ask his doctor for a list of his medications by generic name, in case he needs to obtain some in a foreign country. And, as another emergency precaution, if the patient is taking NPH or Lente insulin, suggest that he take a supply of Regular insulin along as well.

If your patient is traveling where foreign languages are spoken, emphasize that he learn to say (or carry written messages for) such emergency phrases as: "I am a diabetic." "I need a doctor." "May I have a glass of Coca-Cola."

For information about diabetes associations and diabetic care in foreign countries, tell your patient to write to: The International Diabetes Foundation, 3-6 Alfred Place, London, WCIE 7EE, England.

Travel kits for diabetics
On the opposite page are three sample travel kits in which diabetics can carry their insulin, syringes, alcohol, and cotton swabs. The model on the top left is manufactured by Becton, Dickinson and Company (B-D) of Rutherford, N.J. and is made of inexpensive styrofoam which helps maintain a cold temperature. On the top right is a more expensive compact B-D kit, made of plastic. This kit is not insulated and must be refrigerated to keep insulin cold. The bottom kit, an insulated plastic soft pack made by Graham-Field of New Hyde, N.Y., provides room for all a diabetic's needs as well as two freezer packs.

FOREIGN EQUIVALENTS OF ORAL HYPOGLYCEMICS

Orinase (tolbutamide)

Canada	Mobenol, Rastinon, Orinase
Europe	Rastinon, Artosin
France	Dolitol
Israel	Orsinon
Japan	Diabin, Mellitus D
Mexico	Yosulant
Philippines	Oralin

Tolinase (tolazamide)

Canada	Tolanase
Chile	Tolanase
Denmark	Orabetta
England	Tolanase
Germany	Norglycin
Iceland	Tolisan

Diabinese (chlorpropamide)

Denmark	Mellinese
Germany	Chloronase, Diabetoral
Italy	Catanil
Spain	Chlorodiabet

Dymelor (acetohexamide)

Chile	Ordimel
England	Dimelor
Japan	Dimelin
Netherlands	Ordimel
Norway	Ordimel
Sweden	Ordimel

DBI (phenformin)

Australia	Silubin-Buformin, Insural
France	Glucophage-Metformin
Germany	Silubin-Buformin
Iron Curtain Countries	Silubin-Buformin
Latin America	Insural, Inural Retards
New Zealand	Insural
Scandinavia	Dibein
Switzerland	Silubin-Buformin
United Kingdom	Dibotin

Traveling with insulin

Most diabetics are concerned about the stability of their insulin while traveling. They want to know: How long will it be stable outside a refrigerator? When will it start to deteriorate? How will extreme temperatures affect it?

Actually, insulin doesn't have to be kept in a refrigerator, but it should be kept in a cool place. For example, tell your patient not to leave insulin in the glove compartment or trunk of a car out in the hot sun all day. But tell him he *can* carry insulin safely in a handbag or briefcase, or in a suitcase between layers of clothing. If he's flying, emphasize that he should carry insulin *with* him rather than leave it in his luggage, since luggage can get lost or delayed.

Assure your patient that all insulins remain stable for months at temperatures of 68° to 75° F. Specifically, NPH, PZI, and Lente insulins remain stable at room temperature for at least 24 months. Neutral Regular insulin (NRI) remains stable at room temperature for 18 months, but Acid Regular insulin (ARI) may lose up to 25% of its potency at room temperature in 6 months. Insulin stability in temperatures ranging from 75° to 100° F. hasn't been studied, but at 100° F., all insulins lose a significant amount of potency within 1 to 2 months.

Traveling across time zones

Crossing time zones rapidly, as on a jet flight, requires some adjustment in the diabetes management routine. To make the adjustment as smooth as possible, recommend that your patient request a diabetic diet when he makes his flight reservation. And, since eating on time is important, tell him to identify himself as a diabetic to the flight attendants on boarding. If he explains that he must eat at a certain time, they should be able to accommodate him. Of course, he should always carry snacks — peanut butter crackers or hard candy — in case of a delay.

Adjusting insulin dosage also requires some planning. You can help your patient make this adjustment by giving him these tips:

1. Take your usual dose of NPH or Lente insulin, with or without Regular insulin.

2. Keep your watch set according to departure time.

3. If more than 24 hours have elapsed when you arrive at your destination (i.e., if you've traveled from east to west), take a small amount of Regular or intermediate-acting insulin to cover the additional hours gained, *unless* your voided urine specimen is negative. (Consult your doctor beforehand about the exact amount of additional insulin to take.)

4. If less than 24 hours have elapsed when you arrive, take less insulin the following morning. (Again, your doctor will tell you how much less.)

5. After taking insulin in the new time zone, set your watch according to the new time.

6. The following day, take your usual dose of insulin.

7. Follow the same plan (in reverse) on the return trip.

As an extra precaution, recommend that your patient take an antinauseant at least 4 hours before departure time. If he becomes ill despite this precaution, suggest that he take an antiemetic suppository.

If your patient plans to drive extensively, advise him to take 10 Gm of carbohydrate every hour (e.g., an orange, peach, or pear; two graham crackers; or three Life Savers), and to stop frequently and walk around. And, again, suggest that he carry extra snacks to tide him over in case of a breakdown or delay.

Adjusting activities

The diabetic traveler must adjust his activities to his manage-

Have language, will travel

When traveling in foreign countries, a diabetic should learn to say or have written down: "I am a diabetic." "Please get me a doctor." "Sugar or Coca-Cola please."

I am a diabetic.
  French: "Je suis diabétique."
  Spanish: "Yo soy diabético."
  German: "Ich bin zuckerkrank."
  Italian: "Io sono diabetico."

Please get me a doctor.
  French: "Allez chercher un médecin, s'il vous plaît."
  Spanish: "Haga me el favor de llamar al médico."
  German: "Rufen sie bitte einen Arzt."
  Italian: "Per favore chiami un dottore."

Sugar or Coca-Cola, please.
  French: "Sucre ou Coca-Cola, s'il vous plaît."
  Spanish: "Azúcar o un vaso de Cola-Cola, por favor."
  German: "Zucker oder Coca-Cola, bitte."
  Italian: "Succhero o Coca-Cola, per favore."

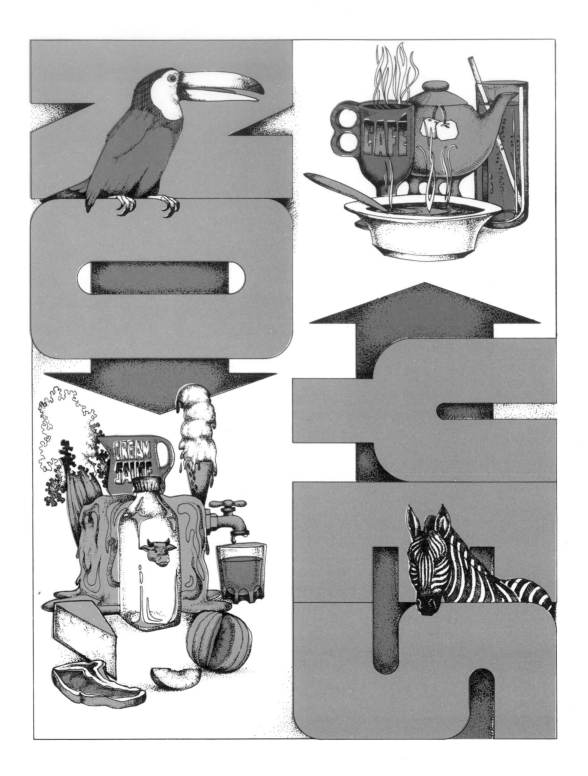

ment routine, too. Urge him to keep up with his regular amount of exercise, but warn him not to overexert himself. Stress that before participating in any strenuous activity or exercise — even sight-seeing — he should either decrease his morning insulin dose by 10% or eat extra carbohydrate (fruit, crackers, or milk).

If he's going skiing, caution him against wearing boots that are too tight around his ankles or legs, since they will impair circulation. If he's going to a beach, remind him never to walk barefoot, even on sand. Advise him to wear sandals to protect his feet against cuts. Remind him, too, to limit the time he spends in the hot sun and to always protect himself against sunburn by applying a screening lotion.

If your patient anticipates doing a lot of walking, he should, of course, wear comfortable shoes. Remind him that even shoes he's worn before can cause problems after walking in them for several hours. Suggest that he pay extra attention to proper foot care. If he develops blisters, warn him not to open them nor to apply adhesive tape directly to his skin. If he must apply Band-Aids, recommend that he use those that have telfa pads.

SKILLCHECK 2

1. Frank Melton, 67 years old, takes 36 units of Semilente insulin every morning. When he brings in his Clinitest results from the previous week, they look like this:

	Day 1	Day 2	Day 3	Day 4	Day 5	Day 6	Day 7
Before breakfast	2	3	4	3	4	3	4
Before lunch	2	1	2	1	1	1	1
Before dinner	trace	0	1	trace	0	trace	trace
Before bedtime snack	3	4	4	3	3	3	3

How would you advise him to change his therapy?

2. Gretchen Hanson, 17 years old, has been taking 30 units U-100 Semilente insulin every morning for about 2 months. At first she controlled her diabetes well. But now she says that she's getting a variable response to therapy. You ask her to decribe her injection techniques. She says she always makes sure she's using a U-100 syringe with her U-100 insulin. Then she shakes the bottle to mix the insulin, wipes the top with an alcohol swab, pulls the plunger out to 30, removes the needle cover, and inserts the needle into the bottle top. She pushes the plunger in, inverts the bottle, pulls the plunger back to 30 units, and withdraws the needle from the bottle. Then she inserts the ½" needle straight into the injection site, checks for blood, and injects the insulin if the needle isn't in a vein. She says, too, that she's very conscientious about rotating injection sites. What is Gretchen doing wrong?

3. Bill Preston, a diabetic who takes 8 units Regular insulin and 32 units NPH every morning, is being sent on a one-week business trip to Paris. His plane leaves around noon Eastern Standard Time (EST) and arrives at 1:20 a.m. Paris time (early

evening EST). Mr. Preston plans to go directly to his hotel from the airport, check in for the night, and get up early the next morning (3 a.m. EST). A week later he'll return on an early morning flight (1:10 a.m. EST) that will arrive home at 10:20 a.m. EST. What adjustments should he make in therapy to account for the change in time zones?

4. Jill Collins has an upset stomach with some diarrhea. She calls you in the afternoon asking what she should do about her therapy. She says she took her usual 500 mg Orinase this morning but, since she doesn't feel like eating, she wonders if she should skip her pill tomorrow. What's your advice?

5. Fifteen-year-old Pat, a brittle diabetic, has had difficulty keeping her diabetes under strict control. But this week she proudly announces that during the past two days her urine tests have read negative before breakfast, at lunch, before dinner, and even at bedtime. What would you tell her?

6. Randy Thomas tells you he's been feeling tired, thirsty, and flushed for the past few afternoons. He says he's taking the right amount of Semilente and Lente insulins and sticking to his dietary therapy, so he can't understand why he feels that way. Because the feeling usually disappears in the early evening, though, he says he's not worried about it. What would you expect Randy's urine tests to show? Would you advise Randy to make any changes in his diabetic therapy?

7. Marvin Kissinger is retiring this year after 40 years of service at his company. As a retirement gift, the company is fulfilling Marvin's lifelong dream — a trip to Germany to visit the cousins he has never met. Marvin was just recently diagnosed as a diabetic. Fortunately, he can control his diabetes with diet alone. But he wonders if he should make any special arrangements for the trip because of his diabetes. What would you tell him?

HOW TO COPE
WITH COMPLICATIONS

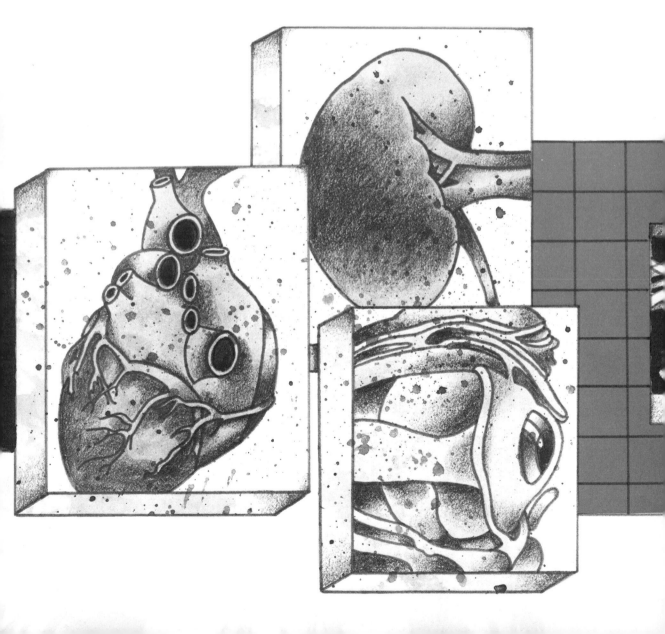

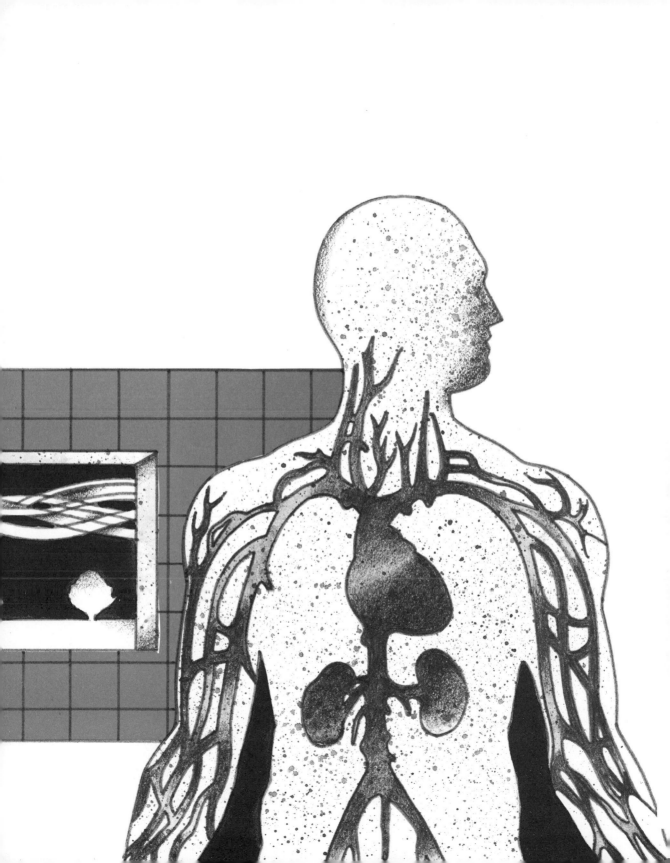

10

MASTERING THE ART OF ASSESSMENT

BY DELORES SCHUMANN, RN, MS

CATARACTS; CARDIOVASCULAR disease; kidney failure; neuropathies of the bladder, eyes, GI tract, hands and feet, and reproductive system; periodontal disease; peripheral vascular disorders; retinopathy; skin lesions and infections; urinary tract infections.... Sound like an excerpt from an index of diseases? It's not. It's a list of *some* of the complications of diabetes mellitus...complications you may be able to help prevent.

The first step to preventive medicine for a diabetic is physical assessment. Which of the many possible ills afflict him? How can he avoid the others? What are the signs and symptoms to look for? How do you answer the questions that worry him, some spoken and some unspoken? How, in brief, can you make your best contribution to the difficult art of managing a diabetic?

Your physical assessment can begin the moment you meet the patient. Note his general appearance and behavior, his clothing and his gait — these can be your first clues to his sensory and motor status. If you shake hands with him, look for atrophy of his hand muscles, an indication of neurological impairment.

Here are other things to examine:

Dermopathy
1. *Shin spots* may be caused by trauma.
2. In about 15% of the patients, *necrobiosis lipoidica diabeticorum* precedes onset of diabetes by two years.
3. *Pyoderma with ulceration* can develop when minor infections are not treated.
4. *Tuberous xanthomas* appear on the buttocks, knees, and elbows; when lipids return to normal level, the xanthomas disappear.

The skin

As you know, the diabetic is easy prey to skin infections. Normally, glucose disappears from the skin at a rate of about 2% per minute; in the diabetic, the rate has slowed to 0.3% per minute. The resulting glucose pool under the epidermis creates an ideal medium for cutaneous infections, especially in the groin, axillae, and inframammary areas.

Particulary in an obese woman can the high moisture and glucose content of skin-to-skin chafing areas support the growth of *Candida albicans*. So, look for signs of that infection: it makes the skin beefy-red to violet-red. The surface oozes, and small pustular lesions surround the clearly defined infected area.

We recently treated a woman in our clinic whose *Candida* infection of the groin had stubbornly resisted treatment. We persuaded her to substitute cotton pants for nylon ones and to stop sitting for long periods on chairs with plastic-covered seats. That worked: her infection cleared up.

Check the shins of your diabetic patient for brown spots — small brown scars with a shallow depression. The brownish color is believed to come from iron-containing substances that remain after small hemorrhages into the skin. The shin is subject to more trauma than most other areas of the body; and therefore the brown spots. The brown spots are harmless, but they are a clue to widespread blood-vessel changes in the diabetic.

Look also for diabetic necrobiosis lipoidica, another lesion seen on the shin; it also results from small-vessel disease. It's reddish-yellow and atrophic, and progresses until it covers a large area of the skin of the lower anterior legs. Despite its appearance, it is harmless.

Watch for pinkish-yellow papules over elbows and knees (xanthomas). They indicate grossly elevated blood fats, especially triglycerides. Although these are not limited to diabetics, they call attention to the continued need for assessing blood fats.

Look especially for skin lesions caused by insulin injection. Fatty accumulation beneath the skin, similar to a lipoma, may form with repeated injection. Patients prefer to use these sites because they tend to become fibrous and insensitive to needle puncture, but insulin will be absorbed poorly from such sites. If you see that your patient needs excessive amounts of insulin

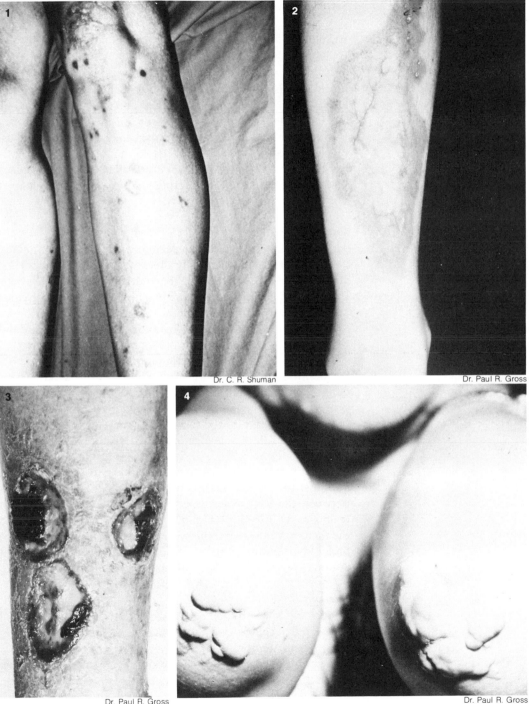

Dr. C. R. Shuman

Dr. Paul R. Gross

Dr. Paul R. Gross

Dr. Paul R. Gross

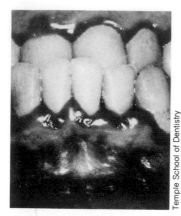

Temple School of Dentistry

Control the diabetes first
In diabetics some conditions won't respond to treatment until the diabetes itself is brought under control. This patient had refractory subacute gingivitis. Since his condition did not respond to therapy, his physicians suspected that he might have diabetes. Once the doctors stabilized his blood sugar with insulin, they were at last able to cure the gingivitis.

to keep his diabetes under control, examine his injection sites to see if they have undergone fatty degeneration.

You may see atrophic areas at the injection sites. Patients are more distressed by these because of their hollowed-out appearance. They, too, are harmless and can be prevented by rotating and distributing injection sites. If the patient has scars at injection sites, suspect improper injection technique — insulin is given subcutaneously at 45° angle. When insulin is injected superficially — that is, intradermally — a wheal raises with each injection. Then scarring follows, as after a smallpox vaccination.

The mouth

The diabetic is susceptible to periodontal disease, commonly called pyorrhea. It eventually destroys the bony supporting structures of the tooth, and the tooth loosens or falls out. Periodontal disease does not always appear as an obvious swelling and bleeding of the gums; sometimes, it goes undetected until the dentist finds substantial bone loss from around the teeth when he probes or looks at the dental X-rays.

Poor oral hygiene and accumulation of dental plaque invite periodontal disease. Dental plaque is a mix of bacteria, food debris, and dead cells deposited from a microscopic layer of protein (called the pellicle) that normally coats all tooth surfaces. If plaque is allowed to accumulate, it hardens, becomes calculus, and then provides a nesting ground for more bacteria.

Teach your patient how to remove this dental plaque daily. He must use dental floss to remove the plaque from spaces between the teeth where the toothbrush doesn't reach, also using proper brushing technique up and down. It is invisible to the naked eye; to see it, the patient must dissolve a disclosing tablet in his mouth to stain the plaque red. His dental care, of course, should be closely supervised by a dentist.

The eyes

The patient's vision should be assessed by recording his visual acuity at each clinic visit and by making a funduscopic examination every 6 months.

He can develop a variety of visual problems. Early in his disease, the diabetic may notice blurred vision, prompting him to ask to have his glasses changed. This blurring may result from fluctuations in glucose levels which distort the lens of the eye. With high blood glucose levels, sorbitol and fructose accumulate in the lens; the lens swells and distorts vision. As blood glucose subsides to normal levels, the lens returns to its original shape, and vision may improve. That is why the patient should wait 6 to 8 weeks after his treatment begins before obtaining new glasses.

Accumulation of fructose and sorbitol can also cause cataracts. The lens swells, fibers deteriorate, and the clefts between the fibers fill up with a proteinaceous substance. The lens becomes milky white and opaque. With the light from a flashlight, you can see the opacity as gray against the black pupil. With the ophthalmoscope, you can see the opacity as gray or black against the red reflex.

Although no one's proved it, chronic simple glaucoma seems to be especially prevalent in the diabetic. Ask your patient whether he has frequent headaches, sees halos around lights, or has impaired peripheral vision, evidenced by colliding with furniture, or, when attempting to cross the street, narrowly avoiding an oncoming car. Look for further clues: a red conjunctiva or a pupil unresponsive to light (fixed in size). Palpate the globe: a hard consistency suggests increased intraocular tension and glaucoma. Peripheral vision can be estimated with the visual confrontation test. The best check for glaucoma, of course, is with the tonometer. When visual abnormalities are suspected, a thorough evaluation should be made by an ophthalmologist.

Retinopathy is by far the most *common* eye problem for the diabetic. Diabetic retinopathy consists of microaneurysms (outpouchings or balloonlike structures on the walls of small retinal vessels) and neovascularization. The new vessels are weak and poorly supported. Serum and blood leak from them because they are so fragile. If a patient has a small hemorrhage from one of these vessels, he may notice "little dark streaks" in his vision. A large area of bleeding appears to him as a red film that blocks his vision completely. These hemorrhages can destroy vision. They may involve not only the retina; they can also rupture into the vitreous. They require a long time for absorption — if they are large enough, they may not be absorbed at all — and scarring follows. The result is markedly impaired vision or blindness.

With the funduscope, check the entire retina, because the

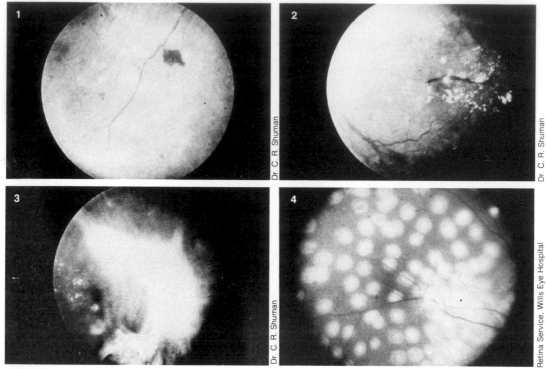

Dr. C. R. Shuman

Dr. C. R. Shuman

Dr. C. R. Shuman

Retina Service, Wills Eye Hospital

Retinopathy

1. *Microaneurysms and hemorrhage* appear as the earliest changes in retinal blood vessels.

2. *Hard exudates, fresh preretinal hemorrhage* (in middle of field), *and neovascularization* appear in the more advanced stages of the disease.

3. With *retinitis proliferans* the patient is frequently considered legally blind.

4. *Photocoagulation,* in this case with an argon laser, can stop the progress of retinopathy.

changes may differ from one part to another. You may notice soft exudates — "cotton wool spots" — where a retinal artery has become occluded and a soft exuding takes place. You may see rings of fluid or serum around microaneurysms, or yellowish blots (known as hard exudates) where this fluid was absorbed but left behind lipid material. Check carefully for dilatation, tortuosity, or irregularity in the caliber of vessels.

Remember that a patient can have retinopathy without visual impairment, which occurs only when the hemorrhage or the exudate involves the macula.

An ophthalmologist must follow the progress of the diabetic who has retinopathy, but you can contribute by making periodic checks of the retina. Although experience is necessary to correctly identify funduscopic features of the diabetic eye, many nurses are acquiring this skill.

The cardiovascular system

Although the diabetic, like the general population, invites heart disease with increased blood pressure, obesity, heavy cigarette smoking, and high blood cholesterol, diabetes itself is among the high-risk factors for arteriosclerotic heart disease.

But evidence strongly suggests that development of vascular lesions can be halted by careful diabetic control consisting of normal blood glucose levels, normal weight, and normal blood lipid levels.

Check the patient's weight and blood pressure systematically. Discuss with him the importance of weight control. As weight is reduced, elevated cholesterol levels decrease slightly, and triglyceride levels substantially. Physical fitness also is believed to help lower triglycerides, so encourage the patient to establish a program to achieve it.

Listen carefully for comments relative to his cardiac status. Does he experience recurrent chest pains, suggesting angina pectoris? Angina pain is produced by exertion and subsides when the activity ceases. The pain is felt in the chest, and sometimes also in the neck, arms, and even the back. Does he take medication for the pain, and to what extent does it relieve the pain? Some patients have chest wall pain not associated with exercise, which arises from structures such as the ribs, nerves, and muscles between the ribs. This pain produces anxiety because it resembles angina pectoris.

The physician may request an electrocardiogram. Remember that a high percentage of patients with angina pectoris and no prior myocardial infarction have a normal EKG at rest.

The peripheral vascular system

A patient with peripheral vascular problems often will tell you he has leg pains that begin when he walks and end when he stops (intermittent claudication). If he has an acute obstruction in a vessel, the pain will persist after he stops. Ordinarily, pain starts in the calf, but, depending on the site of occlusion, it can start in the foot, thigh, hip, or buttocks.

Inspect the legs and feet to judge the competence of circulation. In arterial insufficiency, the extremities are pale, but there is no edema. The skin is cool, shiny, atrophic, and thin-appearing. Nails are thick and ridged, and the patient may tell you that they grow more slowly. There is loss of hair over the dorsum of the foot. Be sure to note the strength of the pedal pulses; in arterial insufficiency, they are decreased, absent, or *"pipe-stem-like."* You can check for arterial competency by elevating the patient's legs 30 cm. Ask him to move his feet up and down; then look for blanching and unusual pallor. After this, have him sit with legs dangling. In about 10 seconds, the

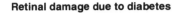

Retinal damage due to diabetes

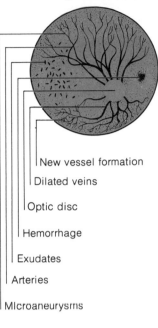

New vessel formation

Dilated veins

Optic disc

Hemorrhage

Exudates

Arteries

Microaneurysms

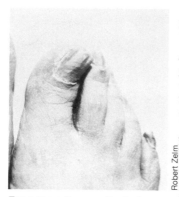

Robert Zelm

Even toenails are affected
As arterial circulation breaks
down, the diabetic's toenails
become thick and ridged and
grow more slowly.

normal color should return to his legs; a dusky rubor that develops slowly is characteristic of arterial insufficiency.

Inspect the legs and feet for ulcerations. With ischemia from the arterial insufficiency, any trauma to the thin, atrophic skin produces ulcers that heal slowly, become a site for infection, and may lead to gangrene.

One man reported to our clinic with a leg ulcer he had been treating himself for some time. When we unwrapped his bandage, we found maggots in the wound. We asked him whether he couldn't feel the maggots. He said no. The fact of the leg ulcer was our first clue that he might be diabetic. His insensitivity to the maggots, because of peripheral neuropathy, was our second. He was later diagnosed as a diabetic.

The kidney and bladder

Kidney disease usually develops gradually. The first signs may be recurring urinary tract infections, or albumin (protein) or pus cells or possibly visible blood in the urine. Symptoms may be intermittent, or absent.

Even with advanced kidney failure, a patient may offer only vague signs and symptoms: feelings of fatigue, easy exhaustion, muscular weakness, and pallor. Because these symptoms are nonspecific, it may be difficult to decide whether to investigate them. Nevertheless, check to see if the patient has noticed swelling of his ankles or face, increased urination at night, generalized itching, bone pain, easy bleeding, or a peculiar odor to his breath. Remember that only a few of these symptoms may be present in the early phases of kidney failure, and they may even occur in relatively good health.

What causes this kidney failure? Diabetes often causes changes in the glomerular capillaries. The basement membrane of the capillaries becomes thick and abnormally porous, allowing protein and red blood cells to pass into the urine. Filtering ability of the kidney is also diminished, allowing waste products to accumulate in the blood.

If the patient is known to have kidney impairment, look for the extent of his edema by checking the pretibial area, the sacrum, ankles and feet, and the conjunctiva. In advanced kidney disease, insulin is not excreted as efficiently, and in effect, its action is prolonged. Check for any *evidences of insulin hypoglycemia.* Also review his program for control of the renal problem. Most often the diet is limited in protein and sodium; vitamins and minerals may be supplemented. He may be taking medication to control blood pressure; review its proper administration with him.

Urinary tract infections are of special concern in the diabetic. As will be discussed in the section on neuropathies, ascending urinary tract infections are common in patients with neurogenic bladders. The diabetic is also prone to a condition called necrotizing papillitis, a result of infection in the renal pyramids associated with vascular disease. Symptoms that occur together in urinary tract infections are frequency and urgency of urination, and dysuria. Besides the symptoms common to UTI, the patient may have a sudden urge to void and lose urine before he can get to the bathroom (urge incontinence). Question him also about possible gross hematuria and nocturia.

Bladder infections in the diabetic may cause pneumaturia — the production of hydrogen gas when bacteria act upon glucose in bladder urine. The voided urine becomes bubbly. Tell the patient about the significance of bubbly urine and advise him, if it occurs, to contact a physician immediately. Should you have an occasion to catheterize a diabetic patient with pneumaturia, removal of the urine is followed by an explosive passage of gas. Pneumaturia is a clue to recurrence of bacterial bladder infections.

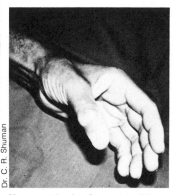

Dr. C. R. Shuman

Neuropathy in the extremities
Patients can suffer atrophy of the interosseous muscle, most marked between the thumb and the index finger. The hands become weak, clumsy, and insensitive to pain. In the feet neuropathy causes the toes to curl up, pulling the metatarsal pads out of place. As the patient walks, blisters form and, without treatment, can develop into ulcers.

Neuropathies

Neuropathy in the diabetic affects many structures and gives rise to a broad range of clinical manifestations, ranging from extraocular muscle palsies to the more common peripheral nerve problems. As you assess a patient's status, be alert to the various areas it can affect. Pay attention to his upper extremities, particularly his hands. Look for atrophy of the small muscles; this is most marked in the interosseal space between the thumb and first finger. Cigarette burns on the fingers or painless burns on the hands acquired while cooking are clues to the extent of sensory impairment. (Blind diabetics have difficulty in mastering Braille because of the impaired sensation of touch.)

Dysfunctions of the extraocular muscles are due most often to impairment of cranial nerves three, four, and six, usually three and six. The first thing you might hear from the patient is that he has a severe pain — a headache, a forehead pain, or an

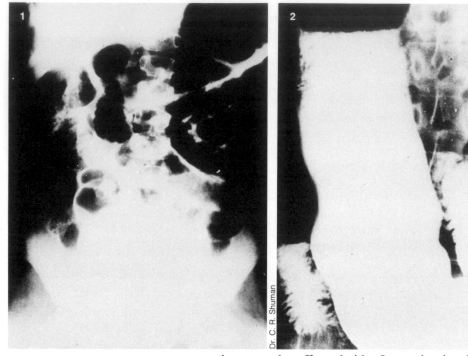

Dr. C. R. Shuman

Gut feelings
1. *Gastrointestinal tract* – Here you will see that the patient's muscle tone has broken down. The emptying of his stomach will be difficult and irregular, impairing control of his diabetes. He may also develop ulcer-like symptoms.
2. *Genitourinary tract* – This diabetic's bladder is severely distended and atonic. As his sensory nerves break down, the autonomic reflex to urinate also deteriorates and he will have trouble voiding, greatly increasing the chance of secondary infection.

eye pain — on the affected side. Later, he develops double vision. Examine the range of the extraocular movements to identify the paresis. Pupil function is not affected. Symptoms disappear spontaneously without treatment.

Gastrointestinal tract. Neuropathy affecting the GI tract gives rise to delayed gastric emptying, symptoms suggesting malabsorption of food, and diarrhea, among others. The diarrhea occurs often enough to merit further attention. Patients complain about intermittent, unpredictable diarrheal attacks that vary in length. They may have alternating periods of constipation and diarrhea. During a diarrheal episode, the stools are most frequent in the late evening, at night, and in the early morning. Stools are brown and watery. Abdominal distress and painful straining do not accompany the diarrhea. Your patient may be embarrassed to discuss his symptoms because of nocturnal fecal incontinence.

Bladder dysfunction. A diabetic is susceptible to neurogenic bladder, often leading to infection, interference with urination, and painless retention of urine in the bladder. He may first notice a bladder problem because of infrequent voiding — perhaps only once or twice a day. He may have a weak stream or dribbling, or he may strain to void the urine. Symptoms can go unrecognized until the abdomen increases in size, suggesting a tumor. A patient may seek medical help because he has symptoms of a bladder infection but is unaware of the actual problem. In a man, the symptoms suggest prostatic hypertrophy.

Reproductive function. Both men and women diabetics experience sexual dysfunction. Although authorities disagree on the etiology of impotence in diabetic men, most believe it is neurogenic. About 50% of diabetic men have organic impotence. They usually retain normal sexual interest, but they notice a slow onset of erectile dysfunction — often described as 50% firm. Masturbation is ineffective in attaining an erection.

What is thought to be the cause? Nerve impairment impedes the transfer of the impulse that causes the penile arteries to dilate, hindering engorgement of blood that is necessary for an erection. This impotence is irreversible; administration of testosterone does not help.

The patient may also experience retrograde ejaculation. He has an orgasm, but there is no ejaculate. Incompetence of the bladder neck allows the seminal fluid to flow back into the bladder instead of being propelled to the outside. Until recently, there was little medical help for this problem. In 1974, one group of researchers used phenylpropanolamine (Ornade) for a diabetic patient with retrograde ejaculation. Semen volume immediately increased, and ejaculation occurred. Following 2 months of treatment, the sperm count, motility, and morphology were normal.

Any male diabetic who seeks help with fertility and sterility problems needs careful examination and counseling to determine whether diabetic impotence is the cause of the problem. Although there is no cure if the impotence arises from diabetic neuropathy, sound explanations to the patient and his spouse can alleviate many anxieties and correct misinformation.

Information about sexual dysfunction in the diabetic female is scanty. Orgasmic difficulties do occur, developing gradually over a period of 6 months to a year after the onset of diabetes mellitus.

Peripheral neuropathy. Peripheral neuropathy affects all extremities, most often the feet and legs. It is bilateral and symmetrical. The patient often is bewildered because he has pain in his legs at night but not during the day. He may tell you

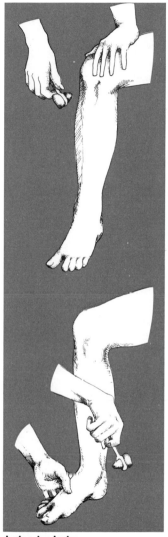

Judge by jerks
To pick up early neuropathy in diabetics, routinely check knee and ankle jerks. With the patient sitting with knees flexed, tap the patellar tendon. Note quadriceps contraction. Dorsiflex the ankle with patient's leg flexed. Tap the Achilles' tendon; watch for plantar flexion of the ankle.

Watch your step!
Diabetics can lose the arch in the
Charcot's joint: the bones
collapse on themselves (1,
opposite page). Note the contrast
with the normal foot on the right.
Because of neuropathies and
circulatory impairment, lesions
and sepsis also can lead to many
serious foot problems such as
gangrene (2) and ischemic ulcers
(3 and 4).

that the pain is not apparent until nighttime; it may not even be present when he goes to bed, but it awakens him during the night. It may disappear again early in the morning. It is relieved by walking. (Remember, pain from arterial insufficiency is intensified by walking.) Question him carefully about paresthesia. Burning, numbness, tingling, itching, or a feeling of walking on cotton or pillows are common. Be alert to the effects of decreased sensation to *high or low* temperature. The patient may have erythematous, blistered, or ulcerated areas because he has used excessive heat to warm his legs and feet. Examine the deep tendon reflexes; in peripheral neuropathy of diabetes, the ankle jerks may be absent.

Lack of sensation in the extremities can lead to bizarre results. A young married woman showed up at our clinic with dozens of peculiar red spots on her hands and forearms. She was being treated for her diabetes. What was this new problem? Skin infection? Rash? Drug reaction? Detective work revealed that she cooked fried eggs for her husband nearly every morning, and never felt the tiny burns she received from spattering grease.

Dr. Max Ellenberg tells of a more gruesome and tragic case involving peripheral neuropathy. A young man lost his leg to gangrene resulting from the complications of diabetes. He purchased a new lawn mower that he could ride around on. One morning, relaxed, he propped his remaining leg up on the machine as he made the rounds of his lawn. He didn't realize that his leg was resting on the hot engine until he smelled burning flesh.

The diabetic foot

Examination of a diabetic is incomplete until you have thoroughly examined the feet and interdigital spaces, and felt the pedal pulses. Neuropathy affects the diabetic foot by causing changes either in the muscle or in the bony structures. The result of the muscular changes is that the toes become "cocked up" or assume a clawing position. This exposes the metatarsal heads. The patient adjusts his gait to the new toe position, forcing foot areas not ordinarily accustomed to the stress of walking to assume it. Calluses form at the metatarsal heads and at sites of walking pressure. Eventually, ulcers develop over these areas.

The result of the bony-structure changes is loss of sensation

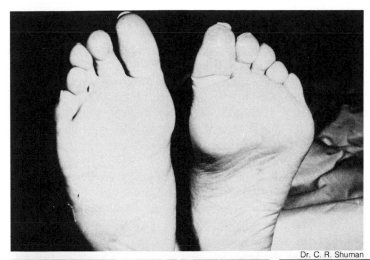

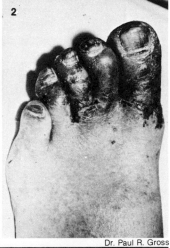

Dr. C. R. Shuman

Dr. Paul R. Gross

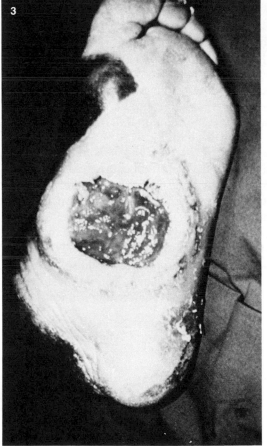

3

Dr. C. R. Shuman

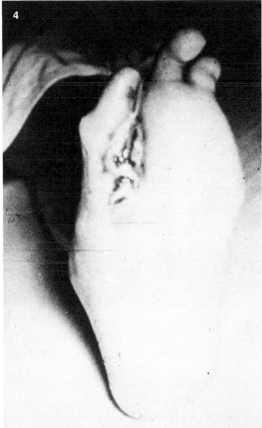

4

Dr. C. R. Shuman

around the joint and relaxation of the supporting tissues. The joint is not buffered as the patient walks, and eventually it becomes jammed. There is swelling but no fluid accumulation. The foot becomes shorter and wider, and the longitudinal arch is completely flattened — it may have a "rocker-bottom" appearance. The patient develops an abnormal gait to compensate for this, again allowing new pressure points and ulcers to develop.

As you inspect the feet, look carefully for neuropathic ulcers. They are usually painless and occur at sites of pressure. Do not neglect the soles of the feet, for the patient may be unaware that an object in his shoe is creating a pressure area. One of our patients developed an ulcer on the bottom of his foot because the heads of two nails protruded on the inside of his shoe. He was oblivious to the ulcer and the nails.

Inspect the feet for calluses. These result from abnormal pressure on the foot, usually from ill-fitting shoes. Once better-fitting shoes are worn, calluses gradually disappear. You can teach your diabetic patient to use an emery board or pumice stone to remove the roughened aspects of the calluses. Trimming calluses to remove the hard keratin and expose the soft keratin should be done by a qualified person such as a podiatrist, physician, or nurse.

Examine the skin of the feet and the nails for evidences of infection. Thick, yellow nails may indicate a fungus infection. Discoloration starts at the open end of the nail and spreads to the nail root. Eventually, the nail begins to separate from the toe and becomes crumbly.

Hardly any organ of the body, from the brain to the toes, is immune from the ravages of diabetes. Because it is a difficult disease to manage, diabetes poses a tremendous educational challenge to its victim. So, the diabetic patient must become an expert on his disease and all its ramifications if he is to learn how to live with it.

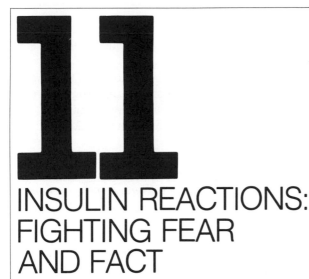

INSULIN REACTIONS: FIGHTING FEAR AND FACT

BY DELORES SCHUMANN, RN, MS

PATIENTS AND PHYSICIANS fear insulin reactions — with good reason. Damage from severe, repeated, and prolonged hypoglycemia can lead to ischemic necrosis of the brain, notably of the vasomotor center. Irreversible damage to neurons can impair intellectual ability and lead to personality changes. In patients with atherosclerosis, insulin reaction may lead to myocardial infarction as well. Retinal hemorrhages commonly appear after an attack.

And yet these are admittedly extremes. For most persons with diabetes, the *fear* of a reaction will fortunately continue to be worse than the reaction itself or its aftereffects. Perhaps the fear shouldn't be dispelled at that. Perhaps it can help you teach the person with diabetes to concentrate on preventing hypoglycemia. In fact, some diabetologists purposely induce a mild reaction so the patient can experience one under safe, controlled conditions.

Of course, abnormally low blood-glucose levels can arrive quite independently of injected insulin. Other possible causes: *Severe liver disease,* which greatly reduces glycogen uptake and release from the liver. *Adrenocortical insufficiency:* here the leading glucocorticoids (cortisol and cortisone) are not present to stimulate gluconeogenesis, in which the liver forms needed carbohydrates from proteins and fat. *An islet-cell*

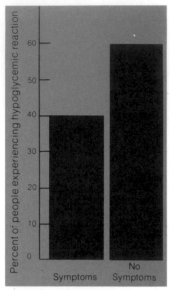

Elusive hypoglycemia
Of the people who have hypoglycemic episodes, more than half experience no warning symptoms. So when teaching patients, stress the importance of testing sugar in their urine on a regular basis.

tumor: by overproducing insulin, this can quickly use up available glucose stores.

Blood glucose can drop, too, when *oral* drugs are used to control diabetes, or when some potentiating drug is given in combination with an oral antidiabetic agent. But here, let's deal only with hypoglycemia from insulin injection.

Not every patient knows
Most diabetics are aware of an oncoming hypoglycemic reaction and can take steps to reverse it. *But a significant number do not recognize premonitory symptoms, and some simply do not display the symptoms.*

Much of our patient education has been geared to the first group, who have an intact sympathetic response, do have symptoms, do recognize them, and do ward off the insulin reaction with food. Even then, too little food or more exercise than usual may alter their response.

For example, after a hard week's work at the office, Betty S., 32, arose one Saturday, took her 40 units of Semilente insulin, ate her usual breakfast, and went off with friends for a morning of tennis. By 1 o'clock, as they returned home, she seemed a little vague and was yawning. Her well-meaning guests, thinking this ordinary fatigue, urged her to take a nap while they prepared lunch. Her husband recognized what was happening and insisted that she drink 4 oz of orange juice. Shortly, she felt nearly normal again.

Her doctor explained that exercise potentiates insulin. So, when she plays weekend tennis now, Mrs. S. cuts her daily dose of insulin (and is not afraid to eat some of her usual emergency roll of candy Life Savers).

Among a second group of puzzling patients are many older people with diabetes who (especially if they have cerebral arteriosclerosis) experience the usual sympathetic response and show the usual symptoms, but seem never to comprehend their meaning. Probably their cerebral function is compromised. Now a slight decline in blood glucose further impairs their ability to reason or recognize their symptoms, let alone cope with them. By the time the bodily adrenergic response releases epinephrine, they are too confused to act on it.

Much of our educational effort should surely aim at trying to make these patients more alert to their own situation. And

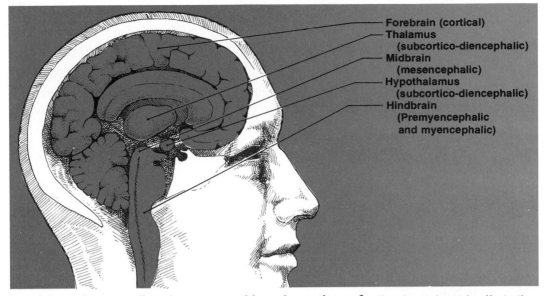

Forebrain (cortical)
Thalamus
   (subcortico-diencephalic)
Midbrain
   (mesencephalic)
Hypothalamus
   (subcortico-diencephalic)
Hindbrain
   (Premyencephalic
   and myencephalic)

certainly, unless they live alone, we could teach members of their family how to perceive initial and prevent further insulin reactions.

Development of a reaction

The symptoms of hypoglycemia reflect glucose deprivation within the brain. Although physiologists once believed that the brain was limited to glucose as a fuel source, we know now that in starvation the brain is able to utilize ketone bodies for energy. Glucose remains its fundamental fuel, all the same. Although many other body tissues store it, the brain has no stored supply of glycogen. So, a continuous supply of glucose has to cross the blood-brain barrier. Any interference in cerebral circulation, say atherosclerosis, worsens symptoms.

Classically, these symptoms unfold progressively as the various brain structures become involved. They occur in reverse order of phylogenesis: the "new" portions of the brain — the cerebral hemispheres and parts of the cerebellum — are the first to suffer from glucose deprivation. These metabolize glucose at the fastest rates.

Lower centers become involved sequentially. The brain structure with the lowest metabolic rate — the medulla oblongata — continues to function long after higher centers have failed. If at last the medulla becomes affected, the patient becomes comatose and obtunded. His breathing and heart rates slow, his temperature drops, his tissue reflexes become

How hypoglycemia affects the brain

The later an area of the brain develops phylogenetically, the greater is its oxygen consumption and need for glucose — and the sooner it is affected by hypoglycemia. Thus the sequence of response is as follows: (1) as the forebrain is affected the patient experiences somnolence, perspiration, hypotonia, and tremor; (2) the thalamus and hypothalamus produce a loss of consciousness, primitive movements such as sucking, grasping, and grimacing, twitches, restlessness, clonic spasms, hyperresponsiveness to pain, tachycardia, erythemia, perspiration, and mydriasis; (3) the midbrain causes tonic spasms, inconjugate ocular deviation, and Babinski reflex; and in the final phase (4) the effect on the hindbrain induces extensor and flexor spasms when the head is turned, deep coma, shallow respiration, bradycardia, miosis, no pupillary reaction to light, hypothermia, atonia, hyporeflexia, and no corneal reflex.

Physiologic response to hypoglycemia

Brain
Drowsiness, loss of consciousness, convulsions, headaches, aphasia, paralysis, twitching, dizziness, depression, blurred vision

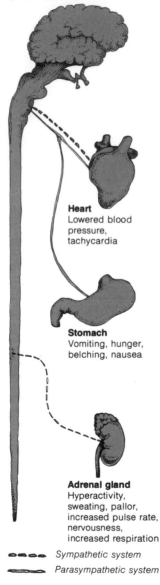

Heart
Lowered blood pressure, tachycardia

Stomach
Vomiting, hunger, belching, nausea

Adrenal gland
Hyperactivity, sweating, pallor, increased pulse rate, nervousness, increased respiration

━●━● *Sympathetic system*

━━━ *Parasympathetic system*

depressed, and his pupils contract and become unresponsive. All reflect medullary involvement.

Some researchers attribute the pace of involvement to varying metabolic needs of the different brain parts. Others now believe the forebrain's more complex neurophysiological connections become depressed by the metabolic insult of glucose deprivation, while the simpler brain stem connections — driven by strong afferent impulses and local chemical stimuli — persist. Either way, glucose deprivation's effects are marked.

Recognizing a reaction

The physiologic response to lowering of blood glucose follows this pattern:

1. The parasympathetic nervous system becomes excited. *Look for hunger, nausea, eructation and possibly slowed pulse and lowered blood pressure.*

2. Cerebral function declines. *Look for lethargy, lassitude, and yawning.* Conversation may become more of an effort. So may simple calculations.

3. In response to need, the sympathetic nervous system releases epinephrine from the adrenal medulla. This stimulates the breakdown of stored liver glycogen into glucose. *Look for sweating, tremor, and cardiac palpitation. Also, look for an increase in blood pressure, heart rate, and respirations.*

During hypoglycemia, this adrenergic response is a valuable one. The liver stores about 75 grams of glycogen to be mobilized; epinephrine is a powerful stimulator of liver glycogenolysis, creating an immediate rise in blood glucose concentration. Epinephrine also arouses the reticular-activating system, so the patient is alert and wakeful. But if liver glycogen becomes exhausted without replenishment of glucose from some source, convulsions and coma will follow.

Yet patients taking long-acting and intermediate insulins may not show these classic symptoms of insulin reaction. With these insulins, the slow decline in blood glucose makes cerebral symptoms more pronounced. There may be change in personality, work performance, or study habits. There may even be aphasia, uncoordinated movements, mental deterioration, or psychotic behavior. The symptoms most nearly resemble alcoholic intoxication and sometimes are mistakenly diagnosed as such.

Another hazard: These insulins often reach their peak of action while the patient is asleep. In the diabetic under stress, look out for nightmares, crying out during sleep, sleepwalking, night sweats, and unusual sleeping postures — all warning signals.

Any misinterpretation delays giving food. And either food by mouth or glucose by injection is the only thing that can ultimately reverse the hypoglycemia and avoid permanent damage.

Assessing a reaction

When the diabetic patient under your care has an insulin reaction, you must assess it thoroughly to try to find its precise cause and also to help the doctor as he determines whether to lower the dose. You will need to know the patient's health history.

Here are several things that can complicate the diabetic's normal insulin-glucose metabolism.

Kidney failure: Ordinarily the kidney degrades and excretes about 7 units of insulin every day. But if the kidneys are severely diseased, less than 0.5 unit of insulin may be excreted. This gives the remaining insulin a longer half-life and in effect raises the dose. Keep this in mind, even when kidney disease has not been established, because diabetic patients are prone to renal pathology.

Liver disease: Diabetes doesn't produce any specific liver disease. But acute viral hepatitis and cirrhosis of the liver are often associated with it. Then, the deficiency of hepatic glycogen makes the insulin-dependent diabetic more sensitive to his insulin dose.

Alcoholism: Everyone knows that some diabetics are also chronic alcoholics. But the combination of injected insulin and excessive alcohol is disastrous. Alcohol prevents gluconeogenesis within the liver; glucose release is inhibited; hypoglycemic coma and irreparable brain damage can result. Since beer and wine contain carbohydrates, the risk with these is lessened.

Medication: Some medications — aspirin in high doses, for example — contribute to insulin hypoglycemia. Find out what drugs the patient is taking and learn which ones have hyperglycemic or hypoglycemic potency. Here are but two:

Aspirin or other salicylates will increase peripheral utilization of glucose and therefore decrease blood glucose. The insulin dose may need to be lowered in an arthritic with diabetes taking large doses of aspirin.

Propranolol (Inderal) is another drug with hypoglycemic potential. This beta adrenergic-blocking agent is used for cardiac conditions. But when the diabetic taking this drug has an insulin reaction, epinephrine cannot act to increase the glucose output from the liver. The stage is set for a reaction without adrenergic defense to buffer it.

Other drugs can produce a hypoglycemic effect, too, by enhancing hypoglycemic reactions or by producing an intrinsic action. These include certain anabolic steroids, guanethedine (Ismelin), MAO inhibitors such as tranylcypromine (Parnate), and certain sulfonamides.

Increased insulin: You should be well acquainted with the Somogyi effect in managing difficulties in diabetes. It works like this: To control rising blood glucose levels, the insulin dose is ordinarily increased. This drops the glucose level, but that in turn calls out epinephrine, adrenal corticosteroids, and growth hormone, all in the body's attempt to oppose the excessive action of the insulin. Epinephrine spurs glycogenolysis in the liver; the corticosteroids stimulate gluconeogenesis. These extra efforts produce rebound hyperglycemia. A doctor, mistaking this for a worsening of the basic diabetes, may inject more insulin and actually aggravate the Somogyi cycle. The appropriate therapy at this stage is to *lower* the insulin dose, and return the diabetes to a stabilized state.

Increasing insulin is a tricky business. When it seems necessary to augment the insulin dose for a diabetic who has been following a satisfactory pattern of control up to this point, be sure that the patient and you, the nurses, coordinate your efforts with those of the physician. Get the patient to record unusual circumstances or symptoms, or any problems, and the times of their occurrence. Sorting and reviewing clues on paper combined with a verbal account make more sense in patient treatment.

A critical misconception
Bill P., a 22-year-old medical student with diabetes, was hospitalized with a kidney infection and had an initial blood glucose reading of 400 mg/100 ml. Additional insulin had brought

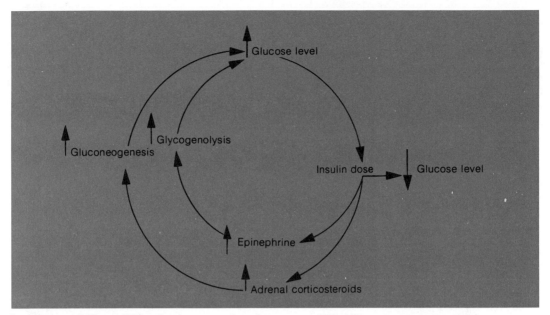

Glucose level

Gluconeogenesis

Glycogenolysis

Insulin dose

Glucose level

Epinephrine

Adrenal corticosteroids

it down to 200 mg/100 ml, almost twice the norm of 90-150 mg/100 ml. Yet the patient was perspiring, trembling, breathing rapidly, and asking for juice to relieve his symptoms. The astute nurse responded to his request, and the symptoms subsided.

Clinical signs don't necessarily correlate with the blood glucose level. Symptoms of hypoglycemia do not depend on an absolute blood sugar reading: they are precipitated by any sudden drop — even from 400 to 200 mg/100 ml.

To get a quick index of blood-glucose level: Put a drop of capillary blood from the patient's fingertip, the earlobe, or a heel puncture on the reagent strip, Dextrostix. Then after following instructions given with the product, compare color reaction on the strip with that on a reference color chart. In any case, this method allows for estimations of blood glucose between 45 and 250 mg/100 ml. But Eyetone Reflectance Meter, a newly marketed product, now has a much wider range of readability for Dextrostix, from 10 to 400 mg/100 ml.

Remember, the diabetic patient whose circulating glucose has dropped sharply will need food or I.V. glucose to avoid the degenerative effects of insulin reaction.

Prevention: how can nurses help?

Be alert for symptoms. Be mindful of how many varieties of response to hypoglycemia there are, and how they vary in the

The Somogyi effect
Some patients who take only one dose of insulin a day have a hypoglycemic reaction by late afternoon only to suffer a rebound hypergycemia the following morning. Increasing the insulin dosage only aggravates the cycle, as this diagram shows. Splitting the same dosage into several injections during the day eliminates the problem and stabilizes the patient's condition.

Hypoglycemia in review

Hypoglycemia is a dangerous condition. Here's a recap of the primary signs and symptoms.

Appearance
  pale
  staggering gait
  delirious
  seizures
  coma
  yawning
  *blanching around nose and
    lips (circum-oral pallor)*

Eyes
  crossed
  dazed
  dilated pupils

Emotional response
  irritable
  anxious
  unexpected behavior changes

Physical response
  trembly
  weak
  drowsy
  cold, clammy sweat
  light-headed
  headache
  difficulty in talking
  mouth and tongue numb

Circulation
  rapid heart beat
  strong pulse

Urine specimen
  *urine negative for sugar by
    second voiding*

Neurological
  Babinski's reflex often present

individual. Teach your patients the more subtle warnings — lassitude, lethargy, hunger, inability to concentrate, to read, to add figures, to think. These early signals are too often mistaken for being tired. But this is when the patient should eat. Help him recognize this.

Keep regular mealtimes. Diabetics and the people closest to them must acknowledge that their actions often set the stage for insulin hypoglycemia. Perhaps you can help them here. To illustrate: Henry P., a 50-year-old businessman, took his 60 units of daily NPH insulin at 8 o'clock one morning. But because he had some abdominal cramping and diarrhea, he didn't eat breakfast. By 10 o'clock he was showing signs of a reaction.

Cheryl M., 19, was trying to crowd too much into a college schedule. She injected her daily morning NPH insulin and ate breakfast. But she didn't finish her lunch because she wanted to get to an exam early. She was unable to complete the exam because her blood sugar dropped too low.

Situations like these should be thoroughly described to the diabetic so he will know to avoid them.

Surprisingly enough, though, hospital routine may be to blame, too. Thomas L., 61, was hospitalized for probable pneumonia and, after his morning insulin, but before breakfast, was hustled off to Diagnostic X-ray. There he waited for 2 hours. He began to feel dull and hungry, and realized he did not have his emergency sugar supply. Just as he was about to go ask for a snack, he was called in for a chest film. He began to shake and perspire. The technician gave him a cup of coffee with sugar. This helped until he returned to his room and breakfast.

Another way we must help the hospitalized patient with diabetes is to bear in mind that his insulin dose may need to be cut as he recovers from a severe illness or from surgery.

Watch out for less food or extra activity. Some patients with diabetes may try to ignore the basic principles of dietary management. You will have first to make sure they understand them. Then explain the importance of adhering to eating quite regularly, amounts, kinds of food, and time of intake. If the requisite food isn't eaten at a main meal, the remaining ration of carbohydrates, proteins, or fats must be substituted immediately. Snacks are also needed to neutralize insulin absorbed at certain hours.

Whenever exercise or heavy activity is planned, the diabetic must either increase his carbohydrate or cut down on his insulin. In an adult it may be best to lower the morning insulin that day. A child should increase his food intake.

Avoid dosage errors. The kinds of errors patients can make in dosage or administration of insulin, leading to a reaction, are too numerous to list. Again, by working with the patient you can help him avoid this.

Be sure the patient knows that insulin comes in three concentrations now. I have encountered patients who, because using the new U-100 insulin means a smaller volume injected than their previous U-40 or U-80, think that they are "not getting enough insulin."

To uncover errors in technique, observe the patient giving himself insulin and checking his own urine for glycosuria at each visit. That's standard practice in many diabetic clinics. I have seen patients misinterpret the urine testing, try to use insulin that has clumped, and mismatch their insulin bottles and boxes. Several times I have found patients reading the unit strength from the box when, in fact, the bottle was of a greater concentration.

Treatment: reversing the symptoms

The initial treatment for insulin-induced hypoglycemia is 10 grams of quick-acting carbohydrate. Overloading with carbohydrate actually slows the reversal and "spikes" the blood-glucose level.

Many people with diabetes restrict themselves to correction with orange juice. Although 4 oz of orange juice contains the requisite 10 grams of CHO and about 6 mEq of potassium, which is also helpful in relieving hypoglycemia, there is no use running around in an emergency to get orange juice when other sweets or sweet drinks are right at hand. The table on page 124 shows several useful foods containing about 10 grams of carbohydrate.

The diabetic should always carry Life Savers, gumdrops, or Space Food Stix or the equivalent in pocket, purse, or glove compartment. But be sure he understands that, though these foods are right for emergencies, they are not to be freely consumed. Children, in particular, are quick to misuse these emergency foods. Some diabetics are better off carrying glucose tablets, marketed as "dextrose tablets" or "dextrose

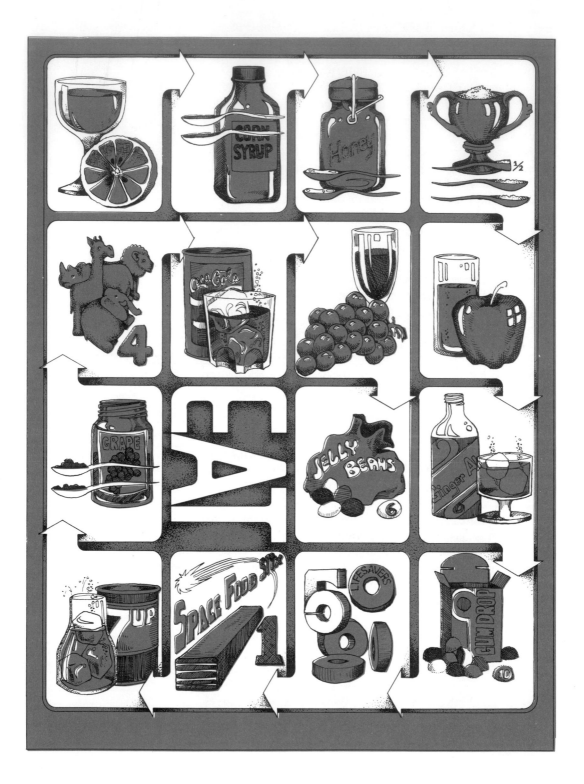

wafers." (These are so sweet they're less tempting than candy.) You might also explain that taking fruit juice when they need sugar gives added nutrients not present in the carbonated drinks and candies.

After the individual has responded to the quick-acting carbohydrate, a *supplemental, slowly digestible carbohydrate must be given*. This will maintain the blood glucose, restore the liver glycogen, and prevent secondary hypoglycemia. Milk, cottage cheese, peanut butter, and bread are good examples.

In severe cases

You can occasionally expect abnormal behavior during an insulin reaction. The person may be agitated. He may spit out food given him. He may spill the juice. But it is unsafe to force food by mouth when his swallowing is impaired: He may aspirate it. Under the circumstances, administering glucagon is the best practice.

This hepatic glycogenolytic substance is produced by the alpha cells of the pancreas. It can be given subcutaneously, intramuscularly, or intravenously. When liver glycogen stores have not been depleted, it will raise the blood glucose in 5 to 20 minutes. If there is delayed response, one or two additional doses can be given. If there is even minimal glycogen in the liver, it should arouse the person enough for you to give him some food until he is seen by a physician. Because glucagon's effects last only an hour, and use the liver stores as well, the patient must have extra carbohydrate.

Every diabetic who is taking insulin should have glucagon available in his home and his family should know how to use it. They need to know when to give it, how to mix it, how to give it, and what to do after it has been given. It is a necessity for individuals who develop insulin reactions without warning.

A second emergency tool is epinephrine, 0.5 ml of a 1:1000 solution (or less than 0.5 ml if it is a small person or a child). This given subcutaneously will stimulate glycogenolysis in the liver, too. But because it also has cardiac effects, it is not safe for everyone.

If the patient hasn't responded to other methods, he needs intravenous glucose. Concentrations of from 10% to 50% are suitable; 50% is most commonly used. The amount required depends on severity of the hypoglycemia. Response is immediate.

How to treat hypoglycemia
The initial treatment for insulin-induced hypoglycemia is 10 grams of quick-acting carbohydrate, such as those shown in the chart. Give 4 ounces of apple juice, orange juice, or ginger ale; 3 ounces of Coca-Cola or 7-Up; or 2 ounces of grape juice. Dry measurements are shown in teaspoons.

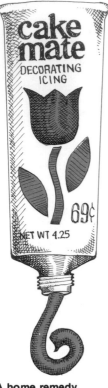

A home remedy
If a patient with hypoglycemia is comatose and you don't have one of the commercial glucose products, you can use Cake Mate Decorating Icing to raise his blood sugar quickly.

Of course, I.V. injection is usually impossible without trained personnel. For emergency use by the family, there are at least three commercial glucose products prepared in a synthetic base with a glue-like consistency. If the diabetic person has a reaction and can't swallow, a prescribed amount is squeezed into the mouth. The solution is either absorbed through oral tissues or swallowed by reflex. Then, as the glucose reaches the blood, he may become aroused enough to take some quick-acting carbohydrate food.

These products are *Glutol, Glutose,* and *Instant Glucose.* They come packaged in plastic squeeze bottles or tubes. Because these resemble medicinals, they should be separately stored, though, where they are instantly available. They are convenient because they are easily given. In an emergency where none of these is available, honey could be used on the tongue in small amounts up to 2 tsps.

And remember
But we should always avoid the suggestion to someone with diabetes that a medicinal is a remedy for insulin injection. His best treatment is prevention. His best protection is a balance among food intake, exercise, and insulin.

If he has a series of frequent, mild reactions, or a single, moderate reaction — or a severe one — he should check with his physician before taking the next dose of insulin. This way, both patient and physician can assess the situation immediately and perhaps adjust the dose. Even if the patient knows how to manage his condition, and knows why a reaction occurred, it is better that he check it out with his physician just the same.

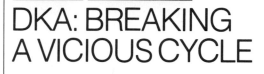

12

DKA: BREAKING A VICIOUS CYCLE

BY DIANA W. GUTHRIE, RN, MSPH, AND
RICHARD A. GUTHRIE, MD

OF THE THOUSANDS OF PATIENTS with diabetes mellitus, all but the most stable ones walk a tightrope. What upsets they face: hypoglycemic shock on one hand, ketoacidosis on the other. Diabetic hypoglycemia was covered fully in the last chapter. Now, let's take a good look at its equally acute metabolic opposite, *ketoacidosis*.

Ketoacidosis arrives by a complex process that may occur in someone newly diabetic, like Donna P. below, or in someone who has had the disease for a long time. It may come on over a period of weeks, or in a few hours if the diabetes was not previously controlled.

With proper treatment this life-threatening problem should be resolved, though, in 12 to 24 hours. Yet even today, deaths are still reported because the illness is usually so acute, because the patient or his family failed to get help in time — or because a really well-trained medical staff wasn't available.

Patient education, then, is critically important. But so is reliable knowledge of the medical and nursing staff who must deal with this problem. You may find yourself taking an active hand in both phases. Do you know how to care for such a patient? The following case tells a typical story:

Donna P., a 22-year-old woman previously in good health, was brought to the emergency room one morning by ambu-

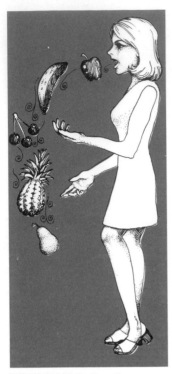

Check for fruity breath
Since the symptoms of DKA and
HHNK are so similar, remember
the one distinguishing sign of
DKA — the presence of acetone.
You can quickly check for acetone
by smelling the patient's breath;
you will smell a sweet fruity odor.

lance. She was comatose, with fast, deep, labored breathing. Her breath had the odor of acetone, and she appeared cachexic. More striking was the look of severe dehydration: her eyes seemed sunken, her mouth dry, and her skin loose. Her sister, who accompanied her, confirmed the doctor's suspicion. Although the patient had eaten with increasing appetite over the past few weeks, she had lost an undetermined amount of weight. The sister also confirmed that the patient had shown unusual thirst for several weeks. She reported that Miss P. had seemed increasingly lethargic and depressed lately...had complained of abdominal pains the evening before and vomited once...and had been found barely conscious this morning.

No urine specimen was obtained, but a blood sample was. To save needed time, the blood was tested for sugar in the emergency room with Dextrostix and for acetone with Acetest. The 400 mg/100 ml plus sugar reading was later confirmed by the laboratory as 500 mg/100 ml. The positive serum acetone reading on the Acetest was confirmed by the lab to be 4.0 mg/100 ml.

What was the diagnosis? The polyphagia and polydipsia spelled early uncontrolled diabetes. The cachexia and the dehydration from polyuria represented its progression. The acetone odor and Kussmaul breathing showed ketoacidosis and the body's attempts to modify it by venting excess carbon dioxide (a chemical breakdown of carbonic acid to carbon dioxide and water) through the lungs. The lethargy, depression, abdominal pain, and vomiting also can go with diabetic ketoacidosis.

Miss P. was given Regular (short-acting) insulin by perfusion at the rate of 5 unit per hour. And she was transferred to the intensive care unit — where these critically ill patients belong — for treatment of DKA.

How did Donna P., until recently a healthy young woman, get to be so ill? Before we review the treatment given her, let's look at the stages of metabolic change that can bring this patient — and others like her — to a critical state.

The road to DKA
Acute insulin deficiency is the cause and the hallmark of diabetic ketoacidosis. When insulin is lacking in blood and tissue, a vicious cycle begins. The absolute lack of insulin

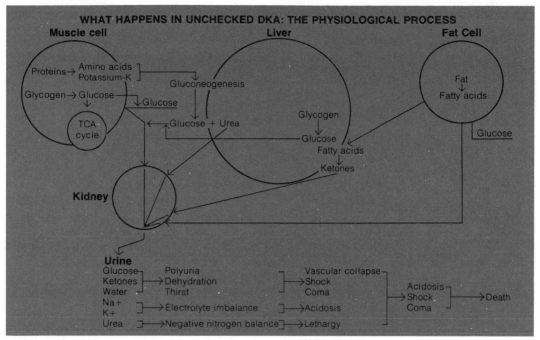

WHAT HAPPENS IN UNCHECKED DKA: THE PHYSIOLOGICAL PROCESS

brings high blood sugar. Although glucose can readily enter nerve tissue, erythrocytes, intestinal mucosa, liver cells, and kidney tubules without it, insulin is essential for the glucose supply of most cells including muscle, fibroblast, mammary glands, the anterior pituitary, the lens of the eye, and the aorta. These cells that need it constitute a large percentage of body mass and energy expenditure, and perform a large part of the tissue building and repair.

Insulin is also needed to facilitate amino acid anabolism for the protein synthesis of cell-building, and to stabilize the storage of fat. Without insulin the body enters a serious catabolic state. It happens thus: Glucose, failing to enter the cells, is not converted to energy but accumulates in the blood. When it exceeds the renal threshold, it spills into the urine. The excess blood glucose becomes an osmotic diuretic; thirst and dehydration follow. So does sodium loss, taking with it some of the body's bicarbonate stores and preventing the needed formation of further bicarbonate. Bicarbonate is the principal blood base for buffering carbonic acid; with its sacrifice, acidosis begins.

At the same time, the cells without glucose are beginning to starve and, so, fats are broken down for energy. Still, they are broken down faster than they can be metabolized. That's

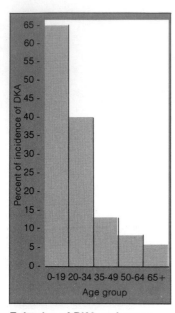

Episodes of DKA and coma
You can see from this graph just
how severe and unstable
juvenile-onset diabetes is. Many
of the young patients suffered
episodes of DKA and coma
because their conditions went
undetected and uncontrolled.
Happily, the DKA fatality rate is
only 3-10%

because insulin no longer suppresses lipase enzymes, and, so, the ketone acids accumulate in the circulation.

The body tries to buffer the mounting acidosis. As the renal mechanism for acid excretion (and bicarbonate conservation) is overwhelmed, the respiratory mechanism takes over. The lungs remove carbonic acid by venting carbon dioxide (H_2CO_3 — $H_2O + CO_2$). So in metabolic acidosis, the respiratory center is stimulated into the rapid Kussmaul respiration characteristic of DKA. As long as this mechanism can compensate for acid accumulation, the pH will not decline sharply and the patient may not seem ill. This may happen even though the 20-1 bicarbonate-carbonic acid ratio will actually shift as serum bicarbonate levels decline. But when the lungs' alkalosis can no longer offset the metabolic acidosis, serum pH drops and symptoms come rapidly.

Protein stores also break down to provide energy to the glucose-deprived cells. But, as with fat, it costs something. The liver, intervening, breaks amino acids into glucose and nitrogen. But without insulin the glucose remains unavailable to the cells and piles up in the blood, intensifying glycosuria, diuresis, and the rest. Nitrogen accumulates, too. BUN levels may rise as urea formation outstrips excretion. And protein breakdown brings marked loss of intracellular potassium, though circulating potassium may be normal or even high.

Many enzyme systems function only within a narrow range of pH. When acidosis depresses their action, the systems — and especially the TCA cycle — slow down more and more. Ketones are less and less well metabolized. Acidosis is enhanced and so is catabolism. The body is now in a state of chronic stress: impose an acute stress upon it, such as an infection, and the patient quickly deteriorates.

Indeed, stress, through its effects of greater adrenocortical steriod output, worsens the existing metabolic alterations. Amino acids cannot be turned into body protein but stimulate the liver to further gluconeogenesis, which breaks them into more glucose and nitrogen. And the glycerol portion of tri-glycerides is set free for further gluconeogenesis; a vicious cycle.

Unless it is interrupted with proper treatment, this cycle of ketosis, acidosis, tissue breakdown, more ketosis, and more acidosis will end in coma and death.

But why the *acute* insulin deficiency? Insulin deficiency is a different matter from adult or stable diabetes mellitus, and has any of several precipitating causes. In early diabetes, the pancreas may actually secrete an excess of insulin. But even in this quantity, it does not exert the same biologic effect for some reason as the same quantity would in the non-diabetic. So there is already a relative insulin lack. Next, though, may develop a progressive insulin deficiency. Again, the etiology is unknown. By now the new and undiagnosed diabetic is in a state of chronic insulin deficiency something like that of the poorly controlled known diabetic. This is what happened to Donna P.

At this point, one of several things may follow: a state of absolute insulin deficiency may be reached. Or, more usually, superimposed stress results in elevated blood sugar, which in turn decreases insulin production. The stress may be emotional trauma, pancreatitis, steroid therapy, Cushing's disease, hemochromatosis, thyroid crisis, or almost any other physical illness; it may be infection, surgery, or pregnancy. Or it may be rapid growth. Or, instead of an insulin deficiency, insulin *resistance* may sharply raise the need for the hormone. Of all these situations, infection and rapid growth are the two most common precipitating causes of DKA. (In the well-insulinized patient, of course, far more stress is required to precipitate acute insulin deficiency than in the one who is chronically insulin-deficient.)

Penalty for stress
Then what was the reason for Donna P.'s sudden acute insulin deficiency? No infection could be found. There was no obvious intercurrent disease, although not all lab reports and studies were in. And the patient, though responding to treatment, was still partly comatose and could not be questioned.

Again, it was her sister who came to the rescue. She recounted that Miss P. had been having a stormy relationship with a man for several months. A few days earlier, after he learned that Miss P. was pregnant with his child, he left for the West Coast with no forwarding address. Donna P., who had obviously been losing a battle with undiagnosed diabetes mellitus for several weeks, possibly because of her pregnancy, was now faced with the emotional upheaval of both pregnancy and desertion. The stress was too much for her, and diabetic ketoacidosis was the result.

Differential diagnosis

How were the staff so sure of the diagnosis? Actually, when all the signs, symptoms, and lab values are put together, little else can be confused with DKA. With insulin deficiency, the first result is hyperglycemia. Only a blood sugar test would pick up this symptomless change. Glycosuria follows, and again only a urinalysis would reveal it. But then come thirst, polyuria, (even up to 3 or 4 gallons a day), and inevitable dehydration, after which oliguria may set in. During polyuria, electrolytes are lost in the urine. As sodium and potassium are lost, there will be muscle weakness, extreme fatigue, and malaise. (Potassium depletion can cause cardiac arrhythmias and arrest. Watch for this problem during treatment as soon as cell repair begins after insulin injection, for it may lower the serum potassium too rapidly.)

With fat now breaking down for energy faster than it can be used, ketones (acetoacetic acid, betahydroxybuteric acid, and acetone) appear in blood and urine. Acidosis begins, with Kussmaul respiration following as a compensation. Acetone's "fruity" odor will be evident on the breath. Often there is abdominal pain simulating acute appendicitis. The cause is unknown, but it may be from electrolyte imbalance and the high fat content of the intestinal tract blood vessels. The patient may vomit, which loses hydrochloric acid, but also sacrifices other electrolytes.

Semi-starvation of the cells now brings hunger and increased food intake, but as many as 20 or 30 pounds may be lost nonetheless. At last the brain can no longer function under severe dehydration, electrolyte imbalance, and acidosis. The untreated patient becomes comatose.

Look for DKA in any patient who is comatose, obviously dehydrated, and in deep labored respiration. Lab values can confirm your suspicions:

— Blood sugar: elevated. Values may range from 200 to more than 2000 mg/100 ml depending upon severity and duration of DKA. Usually between 400-800.

— Serum ketones: elevated usually to 3 or more dilutions of the serum.

— Urine: sugar and acetone both positive.

— Serum lipids: elevated, often giving a creamy, opalescent appearance to the serum.

— Hematocrit: usually elevated from dehydration.

— BUN: usually elevated from tissue destruction and dehydration.

— WBC: usually elevated by dehydration, stress, intercurrent infection.

— Serum sodium: usually low (despite lowered blood volume).

— Serum potassium: low, normal, or elevated — with *body* potassium markedly decreased.

Despite the distinctiveness of these combined signs and symptoms, very often something else may resemble DKA in the beginning. These mimic it most closely:

Renal glycosuria (nondiabetic glycosuria) is free of acetone in the urine. There is no ketosis, and blood sugar will be normal or even low.

Salicylate intoxication may fool you for a while: it can give deep, labored respiration, and a positive urine test for both sugar *and* acetone. But the blood sugar is not usually elevated, although the blood and urine salicylate levels are. Because both salicylate and acetone (ketone) give a positive reading on the ketone test, one can make doubly sure by boiling the urine and retesting it; the acetone of DKA will boil away but the salicylate of aspirin poisoning remains.

Lactic acidosis must be differentiated from DKA, too. Lactic acidosis, though rather rare, is most often seen in the diabetic receiving biguanide therapy (phenformin or DBI). It can also accompany a variety of other metabolic problems, such as salicylate intoxication, ethylene glycol poisoning, methyl alcohol poisoning, paraldehyde poisoning, azotemic renal failure — and even ketoacidosis itself as a coexisting disorder. Except in the last, ketonemia will be minimal but there will be an unmeasured anion, the so-called "anion gap," present in the serum in a value *greater* than the normal 12 mEq/liter. Since the extra anions do not represent ketone, they are probably lactate. Most laboratories do not readily measure lactate and pyruvate. But the anion gap can be figured simply by subtracting from the sodium cation concentration the sum of the chloride and bicarbonate anions, the last determined by measuring the serum CO_2 content. With normal values, it would read, 140 mEq/L serum sodium — (103 mEq/L serum chloride + 25 mEq/L CO_2) = 12 mEq/L unmeasured anions.

When there is underlying disease and you find unexplained

DKA: What to look for
Here's a recap of the signs and symptoms of diabetic ketoacidosis.
— Appearance
flushed face
weight loss
tired
Kussmaul respiration
dry skin
coma

— Eyes
double or blurred vision
soft eyeballs (from dehydration)

— Emotional response
irritable

— Physical response
fruity smelling breath
abdominal cramp
nausea and vomiting
diarrhea
polydipsia (thirst)
polyphagia (hunger)
polyuria (frequent urination)
headache
dyspnea

— Circulation
low blood pressure
weak and rapid pulse

— Urine specimen
urine positive for sugar and acetone

— Neurological
normal or absent reflexes

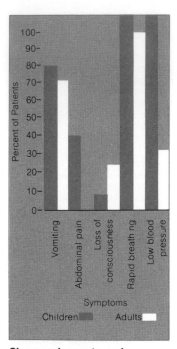

Percent of Patients

Symptoms

Children   Adults

Signs and symptoms in acidosis and coma
Whenever the above signs are present, especially when the patient begins to vomit, consult a physician immediately. Urgency is all the greater when air hunger or unconsciousness appears.

Kussmaul breathing without hyperglycemia and a consequent sharp drop in serum CO_2 and pH, suspect lactic acidosis. This is treated with large amounts of bicarbonate — *never* its normal precursor, lactate. Watch for this condition in any acidotic patient under I.V. therapy, since I.V. fluids often contain lactate. But be especially alert for it in a diabetic who has been receiving phenformin.

Hyperosmolar nonketotic diabetic coma is most often present in diabetics who have been receiving enough insulin to prevent fat breakdown, but not enough to prevent a mounting hyperglycemia, which may run from 600 mg/100 ml to above 1000. The consequent osmotic pressure of the concentrated glucose acts as a diuretic; blood volume is reduced; coma may follow. This diagnosis can be made in a comatose patient who is markedly hyperglycemic and dehydrated, but has little or no ketosis or ketoacidosis. Treatment requires insulin and large amounts of hypotonic fluids, often 10-20 liters in the first 24 hours (see Chapter 13 for more details).

Treatment of DKA
Full-blown DKA is an acute medical emergency. What was the treatment given Donna P.? We mentioned she initially received 2 units per hour of perfused Regular insulin intravenously upon arrival and was transferred to the intensive care unit. In the ER, I.V. fluids of normal saline were also begun to correct the dehydration, sodium depletion, and contracted blood volume. Her treatment in the ICU had these aims:
—clear the serum and urine acetone
—reduce the blood sugar (allowing some hyperglycemia)
—correct the dehydration and electrolyte imbalance.

Some hyperglycemia and glycosuria have to be permitted, lest the patient be thrown into hypoglycemic shock — all too easy. In fact, *the patient can pass from hyperglycemia into insulin shock without regaining consciousness.*

The first laboratory tests ordered for Miss P. and their values appear in the chart on the opposite page. Miss P. was also thoroughly examined for some unsuspected causative infection, and a few appropriate cultures were made. But, as we indicated earlier, no infection was found. The Gravindex test for pregnancy was positive.

Even before the lab results came, I.V. therapy was started to relieve the obvious dehydration. Normal saline as a plasma

TEST RESULTS FOR DONNA P.

	Normal	Initial Value
Blood sugar	60-100 mg/100 ml	500 mg/100 ml (350 mg/100 ml ½ hour post I.V. insulin)
BUN	10-20 mg/100 ml	40/100 ml
CBC		
hemoglobin	12-16	18
hematocrit	33-45%	50%
WBC	5000-10,000	17,500
Serum ketones	negative	Elevated to 4 dil. of serum
pH	7.35-7.45	7.28
Serum electrolytes:		
Na	136-145 mEq/L	128 mEq/L
K	3.5-5.0 mEq/L	5 Eq/L
Cl	100-106 mEq/L	90 mEq/L
Ca	4.5-5.5 mEq/L	5 mEq/L
CO_2	22-32 mEq/L	3 mEq/L
Urinalysis by indwelling catheter:		
specific gravity	1.015-1.025	1.035
pH	5-7	4
reducing sugars	negative	5%
ketone bodies	negative	positive

expander was used initially. Dextran or blood or plasma could also have been used depending on the severity of the vascular collapse. After the lab reported that the blood glucose had dropped to 350 mg/100 ml following the initial insulin dose, 75 units of Regular insulin were given again intravenously. Blood sugar was monitored frequently at the bedside by means of Dextrostix with Eyetone, first every hour; later, as blood glucose values continued to improve, every 2 hours. Results were cross-checked with the lab every few hours. Although the Dextrostix measurement isn't sharply accurate, it will measure the drops in blood glucose that come with therapy. Also, it's convenient when minutes count.

Every hour the urine was tested for sugar with Clinitest and for acetone with Acetest as a guide to further insulin therapy.

Once renal blood flow and urinary output were established, a multielectrolyte solution containing potassium was given through the I.V. catheter. And a cardiac monitor was used to check on its administration. The ICU nurses who looked after

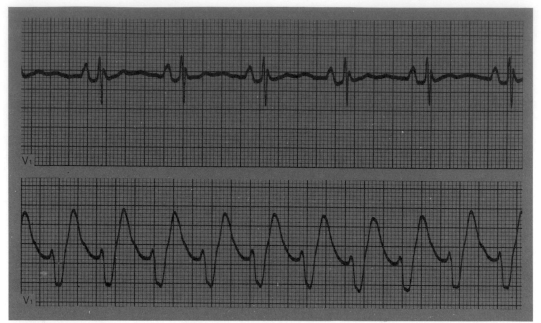

Top — EKG signs of hypokalemia

Bottom — EKG signs of hyperkalemia

Miss P. were trained to recognize the signs of potassium disturbance. (With hyperkalemia, look for tachycardia, then bradycardia; with hypokalemia, arrhythmia.)

It may seem surprising, but glucose was added to the intravenous mixture as soon as blood glucose fell to 300 mg/100 ml. This is done because when insulin is supplied, large amounts of circulating glucose are driven into the cells to be normally used again for energy and repair of tissue. But the blood's stores are small compared to the body's needs (plasma is only 5% of body weight). When the blood sugar comes down to between 400 and 200 mg/100 ml, depending on how high it has been, 5% or 10% glucose should always be added.

The same thing is true of potassium. Once insulin is given, potassium — which has massively shifted out of the cells into the blood and much of that wasted in urine — is then shifted back into the cells again. Moreover, there is a total body deficit of potassium by now even in the hyperkalemic patient. So, with insulin, the serum potassium can drop disastrously. Once the urine is flowing so as to handle the excess, this electrolyte must be given continuously in large amounts. Concentration shouldn't exceed 40 mEq/L, though. And the rate of flow should be adjusted in relation to the serum potassium values or measured by the cardiac monitor.

No bicarbonate was given Donna P. In fact, the use of

bicarbonate therapy in DKA is controversial. Most authorities have routinely used bicarbonate in large amounts to correct the metabolic acidosis. But others have recently questioned this practice, contending that bicarbonate given intravascularly does not cross the blood-brain barrier but rather merely shifts the bicarbonate-carbonic acid ratio. This releases carbon dioxide, which readily *does* cross the blood-brain barrier and re-dissolves in spinal fluid. That raises the carbonic acid level, enhances cerebral acidosis, and may prolong diabetic coma. Correcting underlying metabolic abnormalities with insulin and I.V. fluids containing electrolytes and glucose is sufficient, we feel. Then the kidney and lung will correct acidosis in a more physiologic manner. This problem needs further research.

Insulin therapy in DKA

Insulin is the key to DKA therapy. It should be given as soon as the diagnosis is made. It can be given several ways, and the method also differs for adults and children. *But only Regular insulin should be used,* never the long-acting forms. The delayed action of Lente and NPH insulins makes them ineffective at the time they are needed, and can even make them dangerous later.

For adults, one common method of treating DKA is to give 50-150 units of insulin intravenously. In every case, the size of the dose depends on the size of the patient and the severity of the acidosis. (There is an advantage to I.V. administration: in a severely acidotic patient, hypotension from dehydration is apt to make subcutaneous perfusion poor.) Additional doses of 50-100 units are given hourly until the patient is out of acidosis, then maintenance doses are given every 6 hours subcutaneously. Another method is to begin with 100 units of insulin as a STAT dose, 50 of it I.V. and 50 subcutaneously. In from 2 to 6 hours, subsequent subcutaneous doses of 50/100 units are given, gauged by clinical and lab response.

In children, insulin should be administered on the basis of body weight. Absolute doses may be much too high for small children. Begin therapy with a dose of 1 unit of Regular insulin per pound (2u/Kg) of body weight. Give half I.V. and half under the skin. (Less is given if the ketoacidosis is very mild.) In 2-4 hours, a second dose of ½ unit/pound is given subcutaneously, and in another 2-4 hours, a third subsutaneous

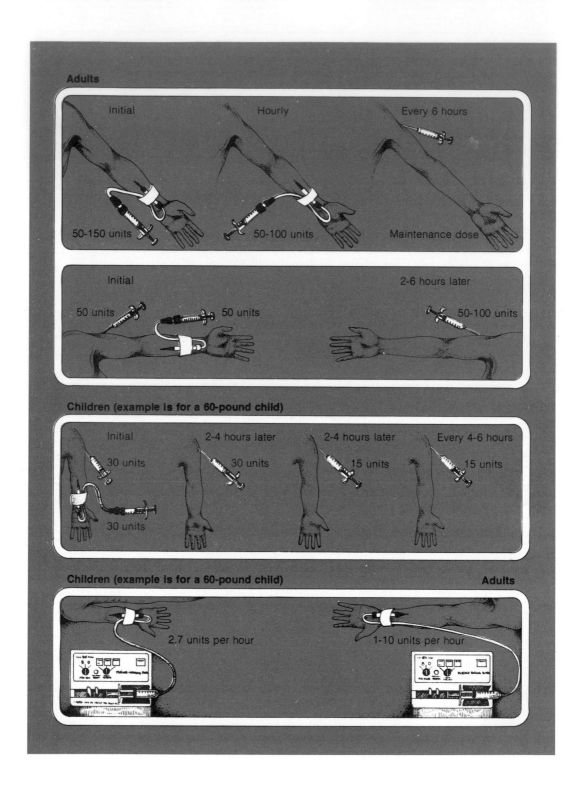

dose of ¼ unit/pound. This is continued with ¼ unit/pound (½u/Kg) every 4-6 hours until the patient is out of acidosis and stabilized.

A newer and safer method involves giving perfused insulin or small doses of continuously administered insulin under regulated pressure ($^1/_{10}$ unit per kilo per hour for children; 1-10 units per hour for adults) until DKA is relieved, as was done in Donna P.'s case. After the perfused insulin is discontinued, blood glucose will rise within 10 minutes.

The doses should always be modified upward or downward depending on clinical response and lab values of the patient. *No rule or lab value can substitute for good clinical judgment.* We find it is always better, too, to underestimate than to overestimate the insulin dose. Smaller, more frequent doses are always safer than larger, less frequent ones.

Initial fluid treatment for DKA uses plasma expanders such as saline, Dextran, plasma albumen, or whole blood. Follow these with "pump priming" solutions of normal saline to expand plasma volume further and establish renal output. Then add potassium and other electrolytes.

Fluid replacements may be calculated in many ways. One of the better ways is to give the patient 2500-3500 cc of fluid per square meter of body surface area/24 hours. Use 2500-up in the mildly dehydrated patient, up to 3500 cc in the severely dehydrated one. These fluids should contain sodium in an amount calculated not only to meet maintenance requirements but to replace deficits. Calculate these by subtracting the actual serum sodium determinants in mEq/L from 140 mEq/L of sodium, the normal value, and multiplying by the sodium space which constitutes about 60% of the body weight in adults and about 70 to 75% in children.

If the patient goes into shock

If the patient passes from hyperglycemia into insulin shock without regaining consciousness, irreparable brain damage may result unless it is recognized and treated promptly. The drug of choice to treat insulin shock or hypoglycemia is 50% glucose intravenously.

Once out of acidosis

When Donna P. came out of acidosis, she was given maintenance insulin every 6 hours. Unless a patient's DKA is very

DKA treatment: how much insulin and when

The drawings on the opposite page illustrate the general treatment for DKA. In the case of adults, an initial insulin dose of 50-150 units should be administered I.V. followed by hourly I.V. doses of 50-100 units. Once the patient's condition has stabilized, a maintenance dose should be given subcutaneously every six hours. An alternative method is to give 50 units I.V. and 50 units subcutaneously as an initial dose and two to six hours later to administer 50-100 units subcutaneously.

With children, the dose of insulin is determined by the child's weight. Using a 60-pound child as an example, an initial dose of 30 units I.V. and 30 units subcutaneously should be followed in two to four hours with 30 units subcutaneously. Two to four hours after that, administer another 15 units subcutaneously and the same dose again every four to six hours after that.

When using infusion pumps, administer 2.7 units per hour to a 60-pound child and 1-10 units per hour to an adult.

mild, the total dose will probably be about ½ to 1 unit per pound (1 to 2u/Kg) per day. Miss P. weighed 108 pounds and her insulin dose was 100 units for the first 48 hours post-acidosis. This was given in 4 equal doses during the first 24 hours after her acid-base balance was restored. When a patient is conscious, this should be accompanied ½ hour after each injection by four equal feedings of simple high-carbohydrate nutrients. In Miss P.'s case, the first two feedings were not given because she remained semicomatose and was supported by intravenous therapy.

In fact, with any of these patients, restoring consciousness may take several hours and should not be a major concern. What is of critical importance, though, is for the ICU nurse to recognize the levels of consciousness and recognize symptoms of hypoglycemia.

After Miss P. did regain full consciousness, her insulin was administered around the meal pattern with 3 meals and 4 doses of Regular insulin. Her physicians later adjusted this to 3 doses (Regular before breakfast, Regular before lunch, and NPH before supper) with 3 meals and a bedtime snack. Before discharge this was changed to 2 doses per day (16 units of NPH and 8 units of Regular insulin ½ hour before breakfast and 6 units of NPH and 6 units of Regular insulin ½ hour before supper) with 3 meals and 3 between-meal snacks. The total daily insulin uptake was adjusted to the previous day's total urine sugar spill.

13

HHNK: INTERCEPTING A "NEW HAZARD"

BY KAREN WITT, RN

HAVE YOU HEARD of HHNK — hyperglycemic hyperosmolar nonketotic coma? It's a newly recognized metabolic derangement, one you may need to recognize to save the lives of certain patients. It can occur as a complication not only of borderline and unrecognized diabetes, but also of a variety of medical and surgical conditions that involve high blood sugar and dehydration. It has *a mortality rate of 60 to 70%*.

Consider the unusual case of Mr. S., who came to our hospital with pancreatic carcinoma. Some months before, Mr. S., age 67, had been found to have elevated blood sugar. Diet had controlled it until about 3 weeks ago, when Mr. S. was brought to the hospital with several complaints characteristic of pancreatic disease, including colicky pain in the upper right abdomen, jaundice, and an aversion to food.

Extensive diagnostic studies indicated a pancreatic tumor obstructing the ductal system. Surgeons did a Whipple procedure. They excised the head of the pancreas along with the encircling loop of duodenum. They anastomosed the common bile duct to the remaining duodenum, similarly fastening the stomach to the jejunum — a pancreatoduodenectomy, choledochoduodenostomy, and gastrojejunostomy, respectively. They left an unresectable tumor around his portal vein.

Mr. S. did fairly well after the operation until late evening of the fourth postop day. He developed aspiration pneumonia with a fever of 101° F. which required Kantrex, Keflin, Solu-Cortef, and supportive respiratory therapy.

By the fifth day his blood gases showed a PaO_2 41 mm Hg, quite below the normal 80-105. Oxygen therapy was started.

Right after the operation, 5% Dextrose in 0.45% saline had been given, to which (when urinary flow had returned) potassium chloride was added. These were to keep the fluid and electrolyte balance normal. Also, he had received 10 units of Regular insulin daily for 2 days; that was changed to 15 units of NPH insulin daily.

Despite the insulin, and although he did not complain of thirst, Mr. S. was polyuric. His I.V. fluid rate was increased.

By the sixth day, Mr. S. was confused, disoriented, and apprehensive. The nurse discovered him hyperventilating with respirations of 36 a minute. He was lethargic, and he looked dehydrated. She found his blood pressure to be only 96/50 mm Hg, his heart rate 130 a minute. Surely by now the classic picture of diabetic ketoacidosis was emerging. *Yet his serum acetone was still zero.* She notified the doctor.

Lab studies at this point indicated a serum glucose of 720 mg/100 ml (far above the normal of 70-120) and serum osmolality of 378 mosmol/kg H_2O (above a norm of 275-295). With blood glucose and serum solutes as high as they were but without acetone, with a pH not acid but indeed a little alkaline — well, what kind of ketoacidosis was this? None at all, as you've surmised. The diagnosis was *hyperglycemic hyperosmolar nonketotic coma.*

On the sixth postop day, Mr. S. had received 4600 cc of intravenous fluid, 1000 cc of it as normal saline during the first 2 hours. On the seventh postop day, he received 6000 cc of I.V. fluids, 1500 cc of half-normal saline with 2.5% fructose and the rest as 5% Dextrose in water.

HHNK is a crisis condition: The first concern is to *restore fluid volume and reduce the blood glucose.* Mr. S. received 50 units of Regular insulin (25 units intravenously and 25 subcutaneously), followed by 25 units every 2 hours until his blood sugar level began to come down. Then he received less frequent doses as he needed them.

Under more ordinary circumstances, fluid replacement would have been given at a rate no faster than 30 to 40 ml/kg to avoid water intoxication — no more than 3200 cc a day for a

		MR. S.'s LAB VALUES						
	Normal	Admission	DPO 5	DPO 6	DPO 7	DPO 9	DPO 10	DPO 12	DPO 13
---	---	---	---	---	---	---	---	---	---
Hematocrit	40-50	42	36			26		40	35
Glucose mg/100 ml	70-120	274	370	720	459	549	460	525	198
Serum acetone	0	0	0	0	0	0	0	0	0
Urine acetone	0	0	0	0	0	0	0	0	0
BUN mg/100 ml	6-21	18		49		59	52	52	49
Sodium mEq/L	134-144		145	164	164	155	151	146	148
Potassium mEq/L	3.5-5.6		4.3	3.7	4.0	3.4	3.0	2.1	3.1
Chloride mEq/L	95-105		112	122	130	121	119	109	108
Total bilirubin mg/100 ml	0.2-0.9	8.6	19.8	14.1	9.7				
Serum osmolality mosmol/kg H_2O	275-295			378	379				
Urine osmolality mosmol/kg H_2O	767-1628			755	810				
Serum albumin GM/100 ml	3.6-5.7	3.6				1.2			
Total protein GM/100 ml	6.6-8.2	6.9	.5	5.1	5.1	4.4	4.6		5.1
PaO_2 mm Hg	80-105		41	75	58			57	57.4
$PaCO_2$	34-46		24.5	22.5	23.9			49.2	44.1
pH	7.35-7.45		7.58	7.53	7.49			7.38	7.38
HCO_3 - mEq/L	22-26		22.2	18.4	17.6			28.1	21.5

man whose preoperative weight was 80 kg (176 lb). But the extreme hyperosmolality and dehydration in HHNK call for extreme measures. So, Mr. S. got a full 10.6 liters in 2 days.

Subcutaneous Regular insulin was being continued according to Mr. S.'s blood-sugar levels. (Insulin added to I.V. solutions can be partially inactivated and, in any case, is supplied far too slowly — unless the patient is in shock, when subcutaneous injection becomes useless because of poor tissue perfusion.) The fructose, which can be phosphorylated in the tissues with no need for insulin, was given for cell energy without adding to the hyperglycemic load.

Mr. S.'s lab values throughout are shown on the accompanying table. On the eighth postop day, his plasma proteins dropped markedly (from 5.1 mg/100 ml to 1.7), so we began giving intravenous albumin. His blood proteins began to climb back toward normal.

A low hematocrit is unusual in patients with HHNK. Mr. S. received 2 units of whole blood because of a hematocrit of 26, caused by loss of blood from his cancer. After the ninth postop day, his blood glucose generally came down a little, too. Mr. S. even appeared to be responding from his hyperosmolar coma. He was more alert and no longer dehydrated.

HHNK: What is it?
The medical and surgical conditions that precipitate HHNK

include those that bring on its forerunner, hyperglycemia: diabetes mellitus, pancreatic disease, pancreatectomy, extensive burns, and glucocorticoid therapy, as well as a variety of acute stress conditions. Like corticoid therapy, the latter lead to hyperglycemia through an overproduction of steroids.

Hyperalimentation therapy has sometimes been a factor in HHNK, and so have hemodialysis and peritoneal dialysis, especially when the dialyzing fluid in the latter has a high glucose content or remains too long. HHNK occurs most often in adults, but occasionally it happens in children, usually from diabetes, sometimes from heat stroke.

To understand just what happens in HHNK, consider the principles of osmolality, or osmotic pressure, that it involves. In osmosis, fluid naturally crosses a membrane to pass from a weaker solution into a more concentrated one. (Fresh water is always drawn into brine.) Various fluid compartments of the body continually establish osmotic equilibrium in this way.

Normally, sodium exerts most of the osmotic pressure in the body's extracellular fluid, and potassium in the intracellular. Still, those solutes that least quickly penetrate cell membranes have the very greatest osmotic pressure, meaning that they most readily draw fluid to themselves, and one of these is glucose. Its molecule is simply too big to get through a cell wall easily. As a result, by remaining where it is, it can attract large shifts of water.

In the pronounced hyperglycemia of HHNK, some of the isotonic intracellular fluid is inevitably drawn out to help equalize the growing osmotic pressure of blood now hypertonic with sugar. Water in the ICF moves out of the cell walls into the bloodstream, after a while leaving the cells themselves shrunken and dehydrated.

Osmosis compromised. But without sufficient water from the outside as well, the HHNK patient's blood becomes yet more concentrated and its volume further depleted. Because, without extra insulin as needed to lower blood glucose, osmotic diuresis takes place.

How? In normal osmolar mechanics, large amounts of body water are reabsorbed from the kidney's distal tubules and collecting ducts. This water, drawn out of the urine that is constantly being formed in the tubules, is restored to the blood: It is extracted by sodium concentrated in the interstitial tissue surrounding the tubules.

But in HHNK, when the plasma osmolality is practically as high as that of these water-absorbing tissues, osmosis cannot draw back the water from the kidney into the blood: There is not a steep enough osmotic gradient. The water is excreted. And the anti-diuretic hormone, though called forth by both hyperosmolality and depleted blood volume, can no longer prevent its loss through tubules whose very means of operating — osmotic pressure — have been cancelled out.

But then something else happens. With this wasting of water, the ensuing hypovolemia decreases renal blood flow. This conserves urine, preserving the remaining extracellular fluid volume. That this oliguria reduces water loss is helpful, but it also severely hampers the kidney's excretion of glucose. Without treatment by insulin and fluids, the process becomes self-perpetuating.

The role of glucocorticoids. Several of the conditions preceding HHNK are often treated with glucocorticoids. But glucocorticoids may even initiate the hyperglycemia (and consequently the water diuresis and so the dehydration) through fostering gluconeogenesis and depressing carbohydrate oxidation, as they are known to do. "Steroid diabetes" may in fact persist for some time after steroids are withdrawn. Glucocorticoids may also inhibit the release of the antidiuretic hormone. And possibly they reduce the capacity of the tubule to reabsorb water and solutes, promoting diuresis yet a third way.

The onset of HHNK is typically insidious, as it was for Mr. S. Once developed, it moves rapidly to a crisis. Early signs in an alert patient usually include polyuria, increased thirst, and a growing impairment of consciousness. Of course, as you are probably thinking, these signs are commonly observed in seriously ill patients of all sorts. And then very often you don't have even these signs to go by because the patients are obtunded or even comatose. But this is why it's medically important to follow susceptible patients closely with frequent determinations of blood glucose and electrolytes.

Failure to recognize the *risk* of HHNK, or to know the syndrome itself when it does come, is bound to contribute to its high mortality rate. But the one big thing about this disor-

Harbingers of HHNK
Usually HHNK coma occurs spontaneously. But it may be precipitated by the following:
   cortisol-type steroids
   phenytoin
   antimetabolites
   diazoxide
   propranolol
   high carbohydrate intake
      in burns
   diuretics such as thiazides,
      chlorthalidone, and
      furosemide.
HHNK can also develop in association with spontaneous Cushing's syndrome and other endocrinopathies.

Terminology

hyperglycemia — more glucose in the blood than normal.

hyperosmolality — abnormal concentration; hyperosmolar blood contains more glucose, electrolytes, or other solutes than normal.

hypovolemia — reduced blood volume; if the patient has not lost blood, he has lost water or shifted it into the cells; the blood is consequently also apt to be hyperosmolar.

osmolality — strength or osmotic effectiveness, written as milliosmoles/kilogram of solvent (mosmol/kg).

osmosis — a natural principle in which a solvent, e.g., water, passes through a membrane from a dilute solution into a more concentrated one.

osmotic diuresis — excessive water loss through the kidneys; an excess of solutes in the renal tubules forces water excretion so as to carry them off.

osmotic gradient — the contrast between the osmolality of one solution and another.

osmotic pressure — the ability of a solution to draw water from another solution across a cell wall, eventually equalizing the concentration of both.

tonicity — osmotic pressure once again, usually expressed as a physiologic norm: A hypotonic solution contains fewer solutes than blood; an isotonic solution contains them equally; and a hypertonic solution is more concentrated than blood.

der that sets it apart from diabetic ketoacidosis (DKA) and other hyperglycemia-related conditions is either *minimal ketoacidosis or none at all.*

If we look more closely at the separate features of the syndrome, we can begin to put it together better.

Hyperglycemia

The most dramatic finding in HHNK is hyperglycemia, linked with the hyperosmolality responsible for coma. Fasting blood sugars may range from 600 mg/100 ml to 3000 mg/100 ml! This high range is usually reached either because of some breakdown in glucose metabolism, or more glucose being supplied to the body than the body can burn.

Clearly there is faulty glucose metabolism in diabetes mellitus and in certain cases of pancreatic dysfunction. In patients with acute pancreatic disease, the curtailed supply of endogenous insulin helps elevate the glucose level. In those with known diabetes, and in those who have undergone a pancreatectomy, receiving too little insulin can be the cause.

In patients with severe infection, or some other acute stress, or receiving glucocorticoids, you will find the blood sugar rising through gluconeogenesis. This synthesis of glucose from protein or fat is a natural effect of the adrenal cortex hormones.

In addition, steroids increase the body's resistance to the action of insulin. With this double-barreled effect in mind, you must be extremely vigilant when glucocorticoids are used with a patient such as Mr. S., or with any patient who may be predisposed to HHNK.

In burn cases, in hemodialysis, in peritoneal dialysis (when high sugar concentrations are used as the dialyzing fluid and remain long enough for the large sugar molecules to be absorbed), as well as in hyperalimentation therapy, patients may receive more glucose than they can metabolize. In hyperalimentation, the prolonged infusion of high glucose concentrations can lead to pancreatic fatigue because of the sharp, continuous demand on the beta cells to produce insulin. If there is at last too little insulin for all the glucose to be used in the tissues, it accumulates in the blood. When the buildup is sufficiently prolonged, the hyperglycemia will lead to actual degenerative changes in the beta cells. Meanwhile, the HHNK syndrome can develop all too quickly if too little supplemental water is given the patient to permit excretion of the glucose by the kidneys: He becomes dehydrated. Be especially wary of dehydration in a patient who cannot complain of thirst.

The blood-glucose level is usually lowered with Regular insulin. Because patients with HHNK are not generally as insulin-resistant as DKA patients, and because there may be severe body fluid derangements, small and probably frequent doses are recommended. But here is one more thing to watch for in these patients whose metabolism has gotten out of hand: their blood glucose level is quite labile. You must monitor them closely, watching a narrow line between soaring sugar levels and insulin shock.

Dehydration and hyperosmolality

No one seems sure whether the dehydration leads to hyperosmolality — high concentration of solutes in the blood — or whether the hyperosmolality dehydrates by causing an osmotic diuresis, as it unmistakably does. No matter which, consider volume depletion and hyperosmolality together as the most serious part of HHNK because they can lead directly to hypovolemic shock.

Under this threat, then, the correction of each one — relieving the dehydration and diluting the hypertonicity of the blood — is the crucial need. Logically, it would seem that hypotonic solutions ought to do the job fastest and best: indeed some authorities have recommended this. Yet it's safe to assume that through osmotic diuresis the patient has lost large total quantities not only of water, but of sodium, potassium, and accompanying anions — despite the probably high serum concentrations of those that remain. Consequently, the use of isotonic saline can help repair these absolute deficits. But, more important, it can do something else: *it can help prevent a shift of water back into the intracellular fluid,* whose relatively high concentration might otherwise withdraw the incoming water from the blood and perpetuate hyperosmolality.

On this basis, here's a three-stage plan for therapy: *Correct the sodium deficit.* The first job is to correct the sodium deficit as rapidly as possible without overshooting the mark — many of these patients are elderly, remember, and may have heart disease. For Mr. S., you will recall, this repair consisted of 1 liter of normal saline over the first 2 hours.

Correct the water deficit. The second job is to correct the

Hydrate at the right rate

Your first and most important step in treating HHNK is to hydrate the patient as quickly as possible. Generally you should use 5% dextrose solution, but remember that a low NaCl concentration must be used with cardiac patients. Use the bottom chart to calculate the rate of flow.

HYDRATING SOLUTIONS

Description	mEq/L	
	Na	Cl
5% Dextrose and 0.33% Sodium Chloride Injection	56	56
2.5% Dextrose and 0.45% Sodium Chloride Injection	77	77
5% Dextrose and 0.45% Sodium Chloride Injection	77	77
5% Dextrose and 0.2% Sodium Chloride Injection	34	34

DOSAGE AND RATE OF ADMINISTRATION (based on 10 drops/cc)

Weight		Approx. Dose	Rate	
lb	kg	ml	ml/min	drop/min
6.6	3	75	1.6	16
8.8	4	90	2.0	20
11.0	5	105	2.3	23
13.2	6	120	2.5	25
15.4	7	135	3.0	30
17.6	8	150	3.5	35
19.8	9	160	3.5	35
22.0	10	175	4.0	40
24.2	11	185	4.0	40
26.4	12	200	4.5	45
33.0	15	230	5.0	50
44.0	20	300	6.5	65
55.0	25	340	7.5	75
66.0	30	375	8.5	85
77.0	35	425	9.5	95
88.0	40	450	10.0	100
99.0	45	500	11.0	110
110.0	50	550	12.0	120
121.0	55	575	13.0	130
132.0	60	600	13.5	135
143.0	65	650	14.0	140
154.0	70	675	15.0	150
165.0	75	700	16.0	160
176.0	80	725	16.0	160
187.0	85	750	16.5	165
198.0	90	775	17.0	170
209.0	95	775	17.0	170
220.0	100	800	17.5	175
231.0	105	825	18.0	180

water deficit rapidly, although incompletely. For *this,* hypotonic fluid is used, rehydrating the patient and yet reducing hyperosmolality faster than added isotonic solution would do. The amount of hypotonic fluid needed by an individual to replace water deficit is based upon a comparison of effective and actual plasma osmolality.

In giving hypotonic solution, you must monitor the serum osmolality to prevent that shift of water back into the cells. Although 0.45% saline alone is often used for the hypotonic I.V. infusion, many physicians prefer fructose 2.5% in saline 0.45% until the blood sugar drops considerably. Fructose is rapidly absorbed from the blood, chiefly by the liver, and so does not contribute either to plasma tonicity or to osmotic diuresis. During the second stage of fluid therapy, Mr. S. received 0.45% saline with 2.5% fructose and 5% dextrose in water.

The third stage of therapy is a *cautious return to normal levels,* including electrolytes. On the eleventh postop day, Mr. S.'s potassium losses were great enough (serum potassium was down to 2.5 mEq/L) to require adding 60 mEq KCl per liter to the I.V., or 120 mEq/day. Of course, the serum electrolyte values don't always tell the true state of bodily derangement. For example, serum potassium levels can be high when the blood has borrowed potassium heavily from the cells, where nearly all of it is stored and used. But the kidneys cannot conserve potassium well. So as soon as the blood's borrowed stores have been partly excreted, the patient will become hypokalemic. By this time, the body may be critically short of its principal electrolyte. Serum potassium levels can also be high in this syndrome when the patient is going into shock, so you should follow these serum values closely in managing the patient. But remember, they're only indicators, not absolutes.

The potassium shift is facilitated by glucocorticoids, either secreted or given. Not only the stress of Mr. S.'s condition, for example, but also the Solu-Cortef that he received must have helped send potassium from cell to serum in the body's effort to keep the latter's levels normal — though they were then lowered by the continuing diuresis of hyperglycemia. Sodium is wasted by the diuresis, too. But proportionately more water is lost, so that Mr. S.'s hypernatremia was primarily a reflection of his dehydration.

Elevated blood urea nitrogen (BUN) is a common finding in patients with HHNK. Mr. S.'s rose after surgery from a normal 18 to the 50s. This increase in serum urea nitrogen comes not only from dehydration but, often, when there is stress or when glucocorticoids are given, from increased protein catabolism. And, incidentally, protein breakdown intensifies the loss of cellular potassium.

Nonketosis

Only the absence of ketoacidosis differentiates HHNK from a regular diabetic coma. When all the signs of DKA are there but this one — particularly when the glucose is elevated — that should alert you immediately to the true diagnosis.

What happens in *DKA* is this: The strongly acid ketones, including acetone, are formed in the liver out of mobilized fat. Normally, after suitable enzyme changes, they are oxidized only for supplemental energy by the tissues and, unless insulin is lacking, they are formed no faster than they can be used. But without insulin (and so with glucose unavailable as energy to the cells), they are called out in force and pile up in the blood as acetoacetic acid, a derivative, faster than coenzyme A can process it.

What happens in *HHNK,* on the other hand, is this: The patient has enough insulin to avoid ketosis, but still too little to reduce the hyperglycemia that is the earmark of this disease. The hyperglycemia, inducing diuresis, produces hyperosmolar blood, but there is no excessive production of ketone bodies and, therefore, no ketoacidosis.

It's also possible, but still speculative, that both glucocorticoids and dehydration have an antiketogenic effect. Glucocorticoids, when given, or when produced by the body under stress, promote the synthesis of glucose from fats or from proteins (along with urea, raising the BUN). But, of course, the glucose without insulin does not nourish the cells; it merely raises the blood sugar, intensifies the diuresis, and heightens the hyperosmolality. The vicious circle closes.

Coma

Coma comes insidiously in HHNK. It seems to be the result of both the dehydration and the hyperosmolarity. Cerebral symptoms are probably due to fluid space and electrolyte derangements. Seizures have been reported during the acute phase of HHNK.

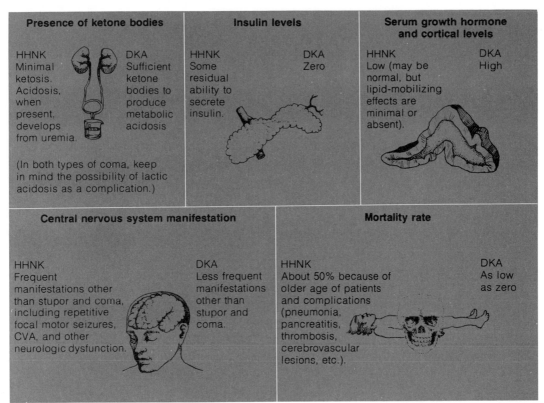

Presence of ketone bodies

HHNK
Minimal ketosis. Acidosis, when present, develops from uremia.

DKA
Sufficient ketone bodies to produce metabolic acidosis

(In both types of coma, keep in mind the possibility of lactic acidosis as a complication.)

Insulin levels

HHNK
Some residual ability to secrete insulin.

DKA
Zero

Serum growth hormone and cortical levels

HHNK
Low (may be normal, but lipid-mobilizing effects are minimal or absent).

DKA
High

Central nervous system manifestation

HHNK
Frequent manifestations other than stupor and coma, including repetitive focal motor seizures, CVA, and other neurologic dysfunction.

DKA
Less frequent manifestations other than stupor and coma.

Mortality rate

HHNK
About 50% because of older age of patients and complications (pneumonia, pancreatitis, thrombosis, cerebrovascular lesions, etc.).

DKA
As low as zero

Nursing care: hydration and sensorium

Here are ways you can help prevent HHNK, and ways to help treat it effectively if it does occur.

—*Know your patient.* Know the pathophysiology of his medical problem. Know which patients are going to run a high *risk* of metabolic coma.

—*Maintain hydration.* To prevent dehydration, record intake and output scrupulously. Record daily weight, preferably on an in-bed scale. Notice the degree of skin turgor and mucosal moistness: Loose skin and dry mouth are both signs of dehydration. Hypotension and tachycardia are *later* signs of dehydration.

You face particular problems with patients who can't complain of thirst, with elderly ones whose sense of thirst is dulled, and with those who are being hyperalimented or tube-fed. Make sure that they get enough water. Usually, it's up to you to assess change and detect need in any of these susceptible patients.

—*And keep a close check on sensorium.* Changes may be subtle. That's why we advise having the same nursing staff

How HHNK compares with DKA
Although initially the symptoms of HHNK seem similar to those of DKA, understanding the basic differences will help you help your patient.

regularly care for the patient — so they can detect change more easily. Lethargy or confusion indicates a hyperosmolar state.

If HHNK does develop, the nursing care plan will be essentially the same, but now the emphasis will be on replacement and rehydration. You must understand the physician's rationale in the plan for fluid administration so you can knowledgeably participate, and monitor progress.

During the first phase, when isotonic fluids are given rather rapidly to replace blood volume and sodium deficits, be sure the venous line is open and the flow rate is as ordered. Watch the vital signs. *Stabilization of blood pressure will indicate restored volume.* During this period, measure urine output frequently.

During the second phase, that of rehydration, when the emphasis is on water replacement and the concern is for fluid overload, you will have to monitor things very closely. The I-Vac can give needed control in the rate of fluid administration. Be sure to check serum osmolality regularly and report any sudden or dramatic decrease to the doctor at once. Again, observe the sensorium. Its sudden deterioration might warn of cerebral edema.

Nursing care: glucose and acetone levels
When you have identified your high-risk patients for HHNK, you can help protect them against it by monitoring the urine for glucose and acetone.

A qualitative measurement of glucose provides the most accurate data. To get it, use a double-voided urine sample — one collected within an hour after the bladder has been emptied. This eliminates your reading any outdated glucose levels that might be present in residual urine.

We use reagent tablets such as Clinitest for glucose and Ketostix for acetone, q.i.d. (Just remember that when the bilirubin is up or the patient is receiving Keflin, you may get a false positive and have to fall back on Tes-Tape or Labstix.) Blood glucose and urine testing should be done on a regular schedule for consistent interpretation of results.

Making the difference
High blood glucose and glycosuria but *no* acetone, or only a trace, and *no* acidosis — these are what separate HHNK from

diabetic ketoacidotic coma. (Lactic acidosis, another acidotic condition that can lead to coma, shows no acetone, either. But like DKA, it produces a low pH reading.)

Treatment differs, too, between HHNK and DKA. In DKA, *insulin* is the key. Smaller amounts of fluid are needed to correct the correspondingly milder hyperosmolality of the blood.

In HHNK, insulin is used sparingly: *water is the key.* Once the lost electrolytes are replaced with normal solutions, the quantities of hypotonic intravenous infusion also needed may bring the total fluids given to *10 or 20 liters during the first 48 hours.* When the hydration problem is solved, insulin may be given more freely.

In fact, giving ample water may easily be the key to preventing this syndrome. All too often, when a patient's metabolic status is fluctuating — not only through imbalances of his own illness, but through the health team's continuous efforts to regulate them — something can go awry. What goes awry to play its part in HHNK is *dehydration.*

Keep constantly on the lookout for it among your susceptible patients — usually the elderly, the debilitated, the mild or even unsuspected diabetic. These are the ones most apt to die. Look to see that their arms and legs are not flabby with newly loose skin, that their face is not pinched and the tongue not dry. Then, too, you should watch for another constant danger: water intoxication. For, as soon as glucose levels are reduced, the hyperosmolality of the blood is sharply reduced. This is when water is apt to be drawn into tissues, especially the brain. *The closest observation is necessary.* Because you are the one constantly on the scene, your observations are most important to the patient. If we are *all* alert to it, a hyperosmolar crisis need not usually develop out of some simple decompensation.

SKILLCHECK 3

1. Frank Masullo has come to the doctor for a check-up. He mentions that he is concerned because he has been spilling sugar in his urine, getting 3+ and 4+ results. Yet he insists that he hasn't made any changes in his insulin, diet, or activity. The doctor checks the injection sites on Frank's arms and thighs. Why does the doctor do that?

2. Edwin Allen, a 72-year-old delegate to a convention, has been found staggering up and down the halls of his hotel at 4:30 in the afternoon. When summoned to the scene, the hotel manager gently offers to show Mr. Allen to his room. Mr. Allen becomes hostile and combative, saying that no one is going to lock him up in "this old folks' home." The manager, assuming that Mr. Allen is drunk, calls the police. They, fortunately, discover Mr. Allen's Med-alert bracelet identifying him as a diabetic and bring him to the emergency room. You find a Med-alert card in Mr. Allen's wallet stating that he takes NPH insulin and has arteriosclerotic heart disease. What would you deduce about Mr. Allen's condition?

3. Margaret Morris has been hospitalized for diabetic ketoacidosis. Her blood glucose on admission was 800 mg/dl, her urine contained ketones and 2% (4+) sugar, and her electrolytes read Na 125 mEq/L, K 6.5 mEq/L, Cl 90 mEq/L, and CO_2 30 mEq/L. Her output is way below normal, her face is flushed, and her blood pressure reads 80/58. What would you expect her treatment to be?

4. Andrew Sims appears in the emergency room with the following symptoms: Fruity smell on breath, flushed face, profuse sweating, strong but slow pulse, dilated pupils, and confusion about where he is. When you check for identification, you discover from his Med-alert bracelet that he is diabetic. What would you expect his diagnosis to be?

5. Jamie, a 2-year-old, was admitted to the pediatric unit with the following: inflamed throat, fever of 100° to 101° for three days, vomiting and anorexia for three days, excessive urination for four days, and polydipsia for one day. His admission blood sugar level was 1720 mg/dl. His urine contained 4+ sugar but no acetone. What kind of crisis has Jamie suffered? What fostered it?

6. Anne Loomis, 25 years old, has just discovered that she has diabetes. When you give her a diet chart, she says she can't read it. She explains that her vision has been blurred recently and that she's afraid she's losing her sight. What would you tell her?

7. Seventy-year-old George Franklin, who has arteriosclerotic heart disease and hypertension, was admitted to the hospital for diagnosis and treatment of extensive skin lesions. The dermatologist prescribed 120 mg oral prednisone daily. Mr. Franklin also is receiving 5% dextrose in water at the rate of 1 liter every 24 hours. After the third day of treatment, Mr. Franklin becomes disoriented; his blood sugar rises to 354 mg/dl. You give him 20 units of Lente insulin, as prescribed by the doctor, but eight hours later Mr. Franklin's blood sugar has climbed to 1340 mg/dl. His urine tests read 4+ for sugar and negative for acetone; serum osmolality is 323 mosmol/kg H_2O. Clearly, Mr. Franklin is experiencing HHNK. What do you think precipitated it?

8. Vicki James, your 18-year-old next-door neighbor, was recently hospitalized and diagnosed as diabetic. She was sent home with a diabetic emergency kit containing glucagon, epinephrine 1:1000 with syringe, dextrose wafers, and Glutose. This afternoon she has appeared at your back door with her kit and says she thinks she's having an insulin reaction. She doesn't know what to use from her kit. What would you advise her?

HOW TO HELP
SPECIAL PATIENTS

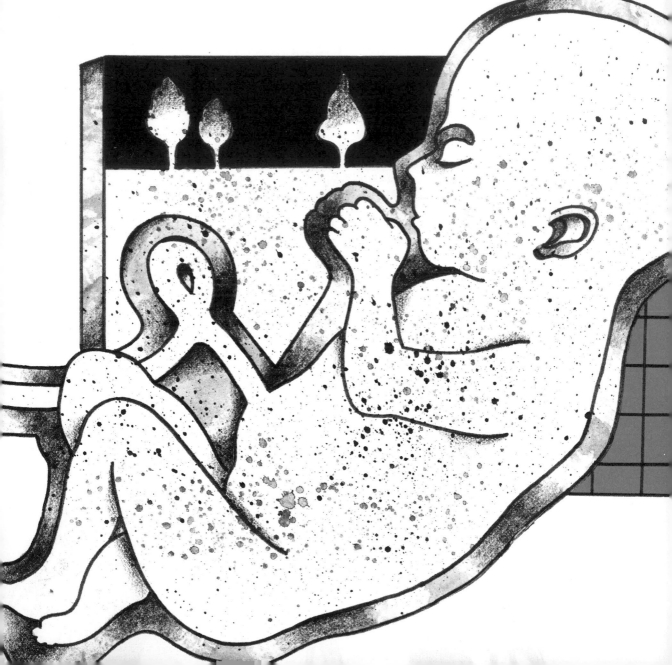

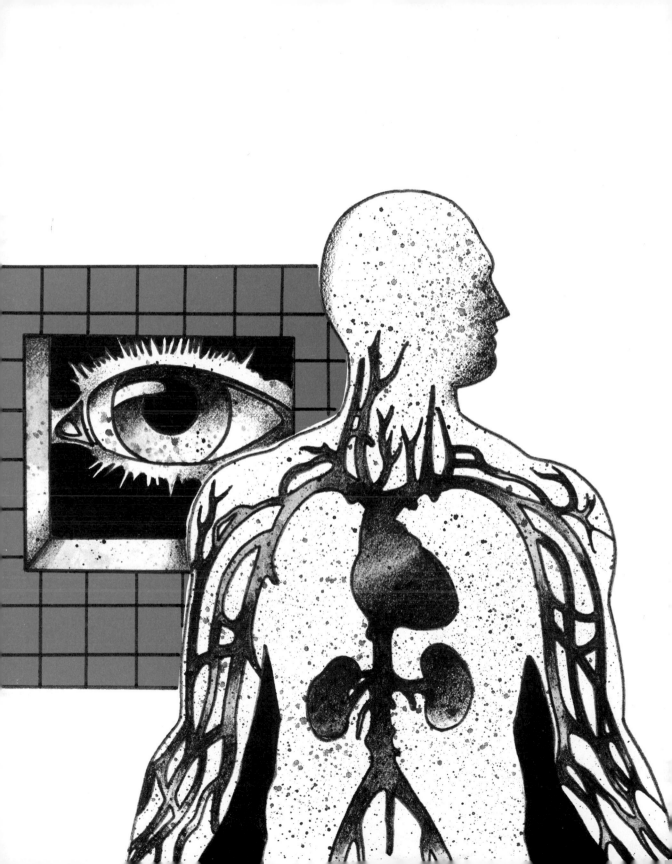

14

DIABETIC CHILDREN: PREPARING THEM TO LIVE

BY DIANA W. GUTHRIE, RN, MSPH

NOBODY NEEDS TO TELL you to manage a diabetic child differently than you would a diabetic adult. The child's age alone and his sure dependency on insulin obviously make his needs different.

But the differences run even deeper than that — all the way to minute modifications in diet and treatment for hypoglycemia to account for the child's size and growth spurts. In short, you've got to manage the diabetic child realistically: As a typical diabetic with some very special needs.

Here at the University of Missouri Medical Center and at the Wichita State University branch of the University of Kansas School of Medicine, we belong to the school of close metabolic control of diabetics. Winegrad and Spiro have shown the need for precise control to avoid later vascular, kidney, and optic-tissue deterioration. Numerous others have shown an inverse correlation between control and early development of vascular disease. No one has proven beyond all doubt that a high level of metabolic control prevents vascular disease or that poor control causes it. But, as of March 1976, the American Diabetes Association stated that a high level of metabolic control will prevent or delay microvascular disease. With this in mind, we continue to attempt 24-hour control of glycemia and complete "insulinization" of the tissues.

Every child with overt diabetes should receive *insulin* as soon as the diagnosis is confirmed. Oral hypoglycemic agents have no place in a child; they eventually only further deplete the pancreas. The child with diabetes probably already secretes little insulin, if any. There is some evidence, however, that giving him insulin early helps restore his own insulin-making ability. The earlier the diagnosis is made, the lower the insulin dose he will need and the easier control will be without hypoglycemia.

The child should be hospitalized during his initial regulation. That enables treating any complications such as infection or ketoacidosis, and also returning him to a good nutritional status. It also enables determining how much insulin he needs for maintenance and educating both him and his parents in his care. If a young patient is undernourished, he may have to stay hospitalized for some weeks.

The untreated child will have depleted his nutritional stores; in the initial phase of therapy he must build them back. This period of metabolic repletion calls for both more insulin and more food than he will later need for maintenance. Once repletion is over with, his insulin requirements will fall back to those needed for energy and growth. His insulin needs may go down to 0.2 to 0.4 units per kg of body weight, or about 5 to 10 units a day. If this "honeymoon period" doesn't occur at all, he may stabilize at about 0.6 to 1.0 unit per kg.

We have found that at least two injections a day of intermediate-acting insulin are the best stabilizing doses for children used to eating normal meals and snacks. In fact, for an adolescent boy in the growth spurt, there is probably no other way to keep him satisfied. With a proportionately smaller stomach in which to contain higher caloric needs, the growing child does best, we find, with three meals and three between-meal snacks.

The nature of the disease
Parents may take it hard at first that their child has diabetes. Better simply explain to them that from now on another part of the child's life chemistry must be outwardly managed just like the eating, drinking, and excretion we are all accustomed to. Let them get over the shock of the diagnosis while helping them all you can. Then go over the steps of the young patient's regimen with them, with the patient himself, and with any

older brothers and sisters who might want to come in on the teaching sessions.

Because juvenile diabetes is fraught with peril, we cannot teach only the care of the syringe and action of insulin. We must spell out what its antagonists are, and what situations call them forth. Such antagonists include hormones like glucocorticoids; catecholamines from stress; glucagon as a natural counteragent produced by the pancreas; and growth and thyroid hormones. Trauma and infection also increase insulin requirement. So do exposure to cold and running a fever. *Exercise decreases it, or else more food must be taken.*

Diabetes is always difficult to regulate when the patient is upset. The adrenal hormones — the catecholamines — sharply increase the need for insulin. But raising the insulin dosage can invite hypoglycemia because the insulin supply may find itself outstripping its counteragents. Then the body will bend all its chemical efforts to raise the blood sugar level through releasing more counteragents. This can set up an insulin resistance that can only be met with more insulin. Hence — a troublesome trip on the physiologic roller coaster that gives juvenile diabetes the name "brittle." Skimping on snacks, increasing exercise, or unwisely increasing insulin can have the same effect if they start the pendulum to swing. Then the child will need a decrease in insulin or redistribution of food intake. Parents should learn to understand when these changes are worth the doctor's attention.

Soon after hospitalization, every child at our hospital receives a diabetic instruction kit containing:
— glucagon
— mixing bottles (if needed)
— variety of insulin (U100)
— vial of diluted fluid for U25 or U50 insulin
— pumice stone, clipper, orange stick, emery boards
— test tube and dropper
— alcohol wipes
— variety of syringes, U100, Lo Dose 50 units of tuberculin (if needed)
— pad of paper, pencil
— identification cards and jewelry
— Clinitest and Acetest
— Tes-Tape
— Clinitest card, 2-drop method

Testing a sibling for diabetes
Have the mother begin the test when the child's bladder is empty. Give a child over 6 years old 8 ounces of orange juice or 4 ounces of grape juice, each with 1 tablespoon of sugar added. Follow it in 20 minutes by 6 ounces of Coke.

Give a child under 6 years one-half the above, except add a full tablespoon of sugar to the fruit juice.

After 2 to 3 hours, have her test the child's urine for sugar by mixing 2 drops of urine to 10 drops of water and 1 Clinitest tablet. Read after 15 seconds, comparing to color-coded card. (If card is not available from salesman, have her use 5 drops of urine to 10 drops of water and 1 Clinitest tablet. Read after 15 seconds, comparing to color code on paper supplied with Clinitest tablet.)

If this carbohydrate load gives the child a positive urine test, the parents should ask the family doctor for additional studies or referral to a diabetes clinic.

Urine testing

Urine testing is easily taught. Still, mistakes are possible, so children should be supervised at least once or twice a week to be sure their technique is correct.

We teach them to use the 2-drop Clinitest, the most accurate sugar-testing method available, and to test for acetone during illness or high-sugar spills with Acetest or Ketostix. They should be shown how to wait 30 seconds for an Acetest to reach its full color by testing a drop of acetone-spiked water. In the Clinitest test they should be taught to keep their eye on the test tube to detect the momentary bright orange (or pass-through phenomenon) that occurs when the sugar is too high for the test to read. Further, if you give the child reasons for it, he's much less apt to touch the tablet, paper, or chemically coated part of the stick. Touching them, of course, can give a false result or even a burn from the caustic tablet.

Insulin

The family may have trouble realizing at first that the twice-daily insulin shot will become as routine as brushing one's teeth. Anyone nervous about the use of the needle can practice on an orange, and indeed the child should. Sometimes to gain a child's confidence, we give the *parent* a "good" injection in front of him and then have the parent use the needle on the nurse. Once parents have given the *nurse* an injection, with a little practice they can give their child his injection, and he will trust them to. We encourage parents to remember they are giving a life-giving medicine rather than fearing they will bungle it.

The younger the child, the longer he will need to learn how to give himself his own shot. Practicing with an orange or a doll helps him work up his courage. Even then, he will probably cautiously try to work the needle through the skin rather than throw it in. But just teach him the basic procedure, and don't pressure him. Soon he will probably ask to give his own medication. We find that imitating his peers in the hospital is one of the strongest motivations. Warn the parents, however, that sooner or later he will give himself an uncomfortable shot at home. Unless they support him he may not want to give himself more for a long time.

We usually give Regular and NPH insulin — two-thirds of the total insulin requirement in the morning, one-third at night.

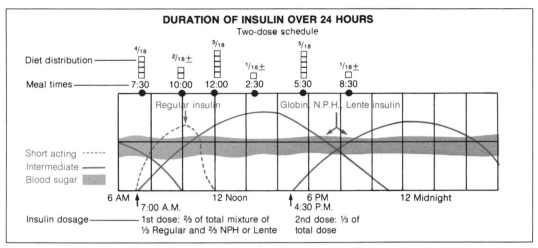

DURATION OF INSULIN OVER 24 HOURS
Two-dose schedule

Diet distribution — $^{4}/_{18}$ $^{2}/_{18}\pm$ $^{5}/_{18}$ $^{1}/_{18}\pm$ $^{5}/_{18}$ $^{1}/_{18}\pm$

Meal times — 7:30 10:00 12:00 2:30 5:30 8:30

Regular insulin   Globin, N.P.H., Lente insulin

Short acting ------
Intermediate ——
Blood sugar ▓▓▓

6 AM 7:00 A.M.   12 Noon   6 PM 4:30 P.M.   12 Midnight

Insulin dosage — 1st dose: ⅔ of total mixture of   2nd dose: ⅓ of
⅓ Regular and ⅔ NPH or Lente   total dose

One part of short-acting Regular insulin along with two parts of the intermediate NPH globin are given first thing in the morning, half an hour before breakfast; the remaining one-third of the dose is given in equal parts of NPH and Regular or, in smaller children, in the same proportion as in the morning, an hour before dinner. (See chart.)

Refinements of the injection technique: Equalizing pressure in both bottles by adding or withdrawing air before drawing the insulin into the syringe; always removing insulin from the same bottle first so that only one bottle will be adulterated by the other, if at all. Because children are so small, an air bubble can displace a significant amount of their insulin daily dose. Show the parents how to invert the syringe so gravity will get the bubbles out. Above all, work out a rotation pattern with them so that the same site will not be injected for at least a couple of weeks. Use a ½" to ⅝" needle so it will penetrate the skin and no further.

If the child shows a patterned sugar spill at the same time each day, teach parents how to change timing of food or insulin or increase the insulin dosage. Infrequent or irregular spills need no change. With more frequent regular spills, either insulin should be increased or diet changed.

Insulin shock
Every parent must be prepared to recognize the first signs of hypoglycemia. Actually, each child seems to feel a little different from every other. The goal is to get him out of it without starting, through overtreatment, the roller coaster effect we have described. Usually a 40-80 calorie increase in food is all

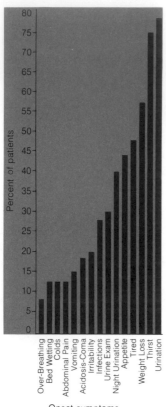

Onset symptoms

Marked onset, quick recognition
Onset symptoms of diabetes appear more frequently and more markedly in children than in adults. As a result, the disease tends to be diagnosed more quickly in children. In the above chart, the results of a study of 513 children with diabetes, you'll see that increased urination and thirst are common symptoms.

that is needed; 1½ to 3 ounces of orange juice will do it rapidly. If the reaction is severe, we recommend giving glucagon — which usually takes 15 to 20 minutes to work. If available, 50% glucose is the drug choice.

In hypoglycemia, convulsions can occur, of course. Parents should be ready to support their child in such an emergency. To warn them of these will add to their concern — but if they are prepared for it, the child will be in safer hands.

Diet management

In all three regimes for insulin administration — 4-dose-per-day, 3-dose, and 2-dose schedules — the patient's calories should be distributed to give him one-third in the morning, one-third in the afternoon, and one-third in the evening. To accommodate differences in short-acting and intermediate-acting insulins, however, we calculate diets in terms of 1/18s of the total calories.

The regimen most frequently used for children at home is 2 doses of insulin. One dose, given one-half hour before breakfast, composes two-thirds of the daily dose. It's a mixture of 2 parts of intermediate-acting insulin and one part of short-acting insulin. The other dose (one-third of the total daily dose) is given ½ hour before supper, and it's usually a 2:1 or 1:1 mixture of intermediate and short-insulin.

To accommodate the varying peak action of the insulin, the child should have his food distributed throughout the day with variation in this distribution related to increased or decreased exercise.

The usual pattern includes 4/18 of the total daily calories for breakfast, one-half hour after the morning injection. The child should eat 2/18 of the total daily calories 2 hours after breakfast. Then, he should eat 5/18 for lunch and 1/18 in midafternoon. Finally, he should eat 5/18 for supper and 1/18 at bedtime. The heavy morning snack could be "traded" for the afternoon or evening snack if increased activity usually occurs at those times. If the exercise pattern differs because of an unusual activity, food over and above the usual dietary plan could be added (or deleted), preferably before the activity (or rest).

The pattern, of course, also conforms generally to that of normal, active, nondiabetic children. They have higher metabolic needs than adults due to their growth. But with a

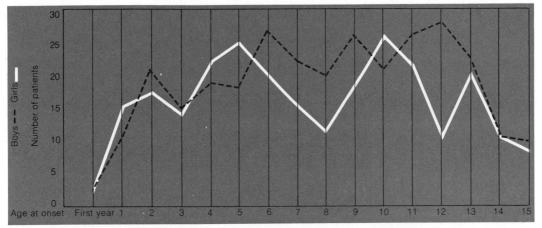

Boys — — Girls ▮ Number of patients

Age at onset — First year 1 2 3 4 5 6 7 8 9 10 11 12 13 14 15

proportionately smaller stomach, they best tolerate three meals and three between-meal snacks. As any mother of a normal adolescent will tell you, there's no other way to keep him satisfied.

During early childhood or the prepubescent growth spurt (or with retarded growth), the child needs 1.5 Gm of protein and 30-35 calories per pound of ideal weight per day. We advise parents closely on composition of this diet, and give them instruction manuals.

Some diabetic diets involve measurements, but we find weighing food easier. It helps train the patient's eye for accurate proportioning. After having weighed food, children can eventually become skilled enough to estimate when they pass through a cafeteria line or are in situations where weighing is not practical. Thus skilled, they can feel freer to travel and choose their own foods. One precaution: the eye tends to "expand" a size, so it pays for parents and child to recheck weights every week or so.

Problems
One of the greatest difficulties will come in relating diet to exercise. If any child is abnormally active, he will need more food. But the child with diabetes absorbs glucose after exercise with less dependence on insulin. Therefore he has got to have extra food, preferably *before* and *during* extra activity. Trial and error must determine if it is the right amount, judged by whether sugar is spilled in the urine, or symptoms of hypoglycemia come on.

We encourage parents to work toward two goals: when the child is well, to keep his urine as free of sugar as possible

Age at onset
In children, the average age of diabetes onset seems to be eight years, according to a study of 600 juvenile-onset diabetics. Diabetes occurs as often in boys as in girls.

without his experiencing an insulin reaction; when he is ill, to keep his urine sugar down to less than 2% (4+) and be free of acetone. Everything is recorded: 3 to 4 daily urine tests for sugar, acetone when needed, the time, kind and amounts of insulin injection, reactions, diet changes, exercise, everything. When accurate records are kept, danger signs show up. The doctor may have to increase the insulin whenever a cold or other infection strikes to keep it from making the child needlessly ill. Parents should know when to call.

Money is usually a problem in any chronic illness. If the parents know beforehand how much supplies and insulin cost, they will start to budget for future needs. Most of all, the child should be hospitalized long enough for him and his parents to be really well trained in managing his illness. A number of studies have determined that the more parents and families know about handling diabetes, the less hospitalization is needed later one. Perhaps this first time will be the only hospitalization a child will ever have for his metabolic flaw.

A child will learn best in short sessions — say 15 to 20 minutes or even less. The parents do best in periods of 45 to 60 minutes or even longer if they are inquisitive. We always review the previous day's instruction to bring out questions or problems. And we depend heavily on films, filmstrips, pictures, articles, and manuals.

We try to encourage parents and children to think of diabetes as a challenge to face rather than a problem to hide. We tell the children to wear identification for self-protection. We tell them to follow the regimen, but go ahead trick or treating, or whatever, with the other kids. We tell them not to think of it as "I can't eat that candy," but simply as "Who would I like to share with?" By the time a child is 9 or 10 he should be able to manage his regimen himself under supervision.

We stress that the more active the child is, the more manageable his diabetes will be. And activity has other advantages. The person with well-controlled diabetes is becoming known as a better employment risk than the average. In fact, some of the greatest people in the world have had to overcome handicaps. With all their self-discipline, there's a lot these initiates can do. And you — the nurse who teaches early — can make the difference between disability and victory.

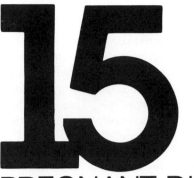

15

PREGNANT DIABETICS: DISPELLING MYTHS

BY CATHERINE GAROFANO, RN, BS

CONTEMPLATING MOTHERHOOD can be worrisome for any woman — especially if she lacks adequate prenatal instruction. For the diabetic, it's doubly so. That's why it's so important that every nurse who works with pregnant diabetics understand their unique problems.

Like most other women, a diabetic may be concerned about her emotional fitness for motherhood. But unlike most other women, she'll probably be more concerned about her *physical* fitness. Can she conceive? Would pregnancy adversely affect her diabetes? Would her diabetes harm her baby?

Confronted with these enormous concerns, she may turn to you with the unsettling question: "Should I have a baby?" Of course, you can't and shouldn't answer that question for her. But by separating the myths about diabetic pregnancy from the realities, you can help her and her husband answer it themselves.

Following are some common concerns and helpful answers. Before you get into these, read the chart on page 169. It explains diabetes-specialist Dr. Priscilla White's classification of diabetes according to onset and severity of disease. This widely used classification system will help you advise a diabetic woman on which complications, both fetal and maternal, she can anticipate during pregnancy.

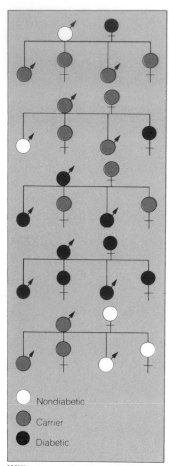

Nondiabetic

Carrier

Diabetic

Will your patient's child have diabetes?
Based on Mendelian statistics, the chances of a child developing diabetes would be as above. But these statistics are still indefinite since no one knows the exact relationship between heredity and diabetes. Recent studies suggest that the genetic factor is lower than once thought.

"Will I have trouble getting pregnant?"

Before insulin became available, the answer would have been an unqualified "yes." Few juvenile-onset diabetics lived to adulthood; many of those who did were sterile. Today, though, the answer is almost always "no." Usually only the most severely diabetic women or those with uncontrolled diabetes have trouble getting pregnant.

"Would I transmit diabetes to my baby?"

While it's true that diabetes has some genetic component, the risk of transmittal isn't as great as once thought. In fact, some statistics suggest that the child of a diabetic parent has as little as a 1% chance of developing diabetes before age 10. The risk increases with age. But the same statistics suggest that, even at age 60, the offspring of a diabetic parent still has only a 10% chance of developing diabetes. These percentages apply whether the mother or father is diabetic. If both are diabetic, though, the percentages double.

"Would the baby have more problems than the child of a normal mother?"

Perhaps. Babies of diabetic mothers tend to be heavier, often more than 9 pounds — especially if the mother develops diabetes during pregnancy (gestational diabetes) or is a Class A or Class B diabetic (as defined in the accompanying chart). Despite their heavy birth weight, they tend to be immature and are more likely to develop respiratory distress syndrome. Fortunately, though, this complication has been waning recently due to the development of indices that allow the doctor to select the best time for delivery.

Babies of diabetic fathers don't run any greater risk of congenital anomalies than babies of normal parents. But babies of diabetic mothers run twice the risk (about 13% compared to 6% for the general population). Among these anomalies: cardiac malformations, brain damage due to cerebral hemorrhage, traumatic birth due to the baby's large size, hypocalcemia or hyperbilirubinemia, and hypoglycemia. Hypoglycemia used to be a common cause of neonatal death, but today doctors can recognize it early and treat it promptly with glucose infusions. Today, neonatal deaths among diabetic women run only about 10%, compared to 3% for the general population.

"Would I have more trouble with pregnancy than a nondiabetic woman? Would pregnancy make my diabetes worse?"

The effects of pregnancy all depend on the mother's condition. Pregnancy itself is an "insulin antagonistic state." That means a woman needs more insulin to maintain normal carbohydrate metabolism during pregnancy. A normal person can meet that demand easily, but a woman with diabetes or a tendency toward diabetes can't. Her carbohydrate metabolism deteriorates, resulting in mild to severe hyperglycemia and even ketoacidosis if not adequately treated with insulin.

Pregnant diabetics are more likely than nondiabetics to suffer from the following: hydramnios, toxemia, and urinary tract infections. Hydramnios, an excess of amniotic fluid, appears to some degree in about 20% of all pregnant diabetics. With judicious use of diuretics, though, doctors can prevent hydramnios from prematurely rupturing membranes. Diabetics also are five times more prone to toxemia with proteinuria, hypertension, and edema than the general population. There is an increased incidence of urinary tract infections that may adversely affect pregnancy. But these urinary tract infections usually respond quite well to medical therapy.

Besides these problems, 10% of Class R diabetics may have progression of the disease to serious visual impairment or blindness. Most Class F diabetics have renal deterioration. But generally, renal function returns to its pre-pregnant state after delivery. If a woman is threatened by these complications, she and her doctor will have to decide whether she should avoid or interrupt pregnancy.

"Would I go into labor normally and deliver vaginally? Or would I be delivered early or have a cesarean section?"

That depends on the mother's type of diabetes, her condition during pregnancy, and the baby's condition.

THE COURSE OF PREGNANCY BY CLASS

Complication	A	B	C	D	F	R
spontaneous abortion rate	N	N	N	+	++++	++++
hydramnios degree	+	++++	+++	++	±	±
excessive maternal weight gain	+	++++	+++	++	0	0
toxemia, i.e., preclampsia	+	++++	+++	++	?	superimposed?
large placenta	+++	++++	+++	++	0	0
heavy-birth-weight infant	++++	++++	+++	++	0	0
intrauterine fetal loss	+	++	+	+++	++++	++++
intrapartum fetal loss	++++	++++	++	+	+	+
neonatal loss	+	+	++	+++	++++	++++
congenital abnormalities	+	+	+	+	++	+++
diabetes mellitus intensified	+	++++	+++	+	±	±

Legend

N - *Normal*

? – *hard to tell*

+ - *minimal chance*
++++ - *maximum chance*

super-imposed-patient already had symptoms which are possibly extenuated

0 - *not significant*

± - *the condition is possible*

If a woman is a Class A diabetic, the doctor will check her condition and the baby's size often, especially a week before the expected due date. If everything seems okay, he may allow her to go into spontaneous labor with a normal vaginal delivery. If he has any question about the expected delivery date, he'll usually induce labor somewhere during the 38th, 39th, or 40th week for a normal vaginal delivery. If pregnancy runs beyond the 40th week, he'll induce labor.

If a woman is a Class B or C diabetic, the doctor probably will induce labor during the 36th or 37th week. If she's a Class D, F, or R diabetic, he'll probably hospitalize her 6 to 8 weeks before her expected due date. And, unless she needs an emergency delivery at some earlier time, he'll induce labor during the 35th or 36th week. In every case, he'll order chemical tests to determine the very best time for delivery.

If at all possible, most doctors prefer a vaginal delivery. But if the mother runs into complications such as toxemia, if the fetus shows signs of distress, or if the fetus is too large for an easy vaginal delivery, the doctor will perform a cesarean section.

"You said the doctor will determine the best time for delivery. How can he do that?"

With the help of a few simple tests.

First, he'll check the estriol level in the mother's urine or blood. A decrease in the estriol level indicates a failing placenta and may signal the need for immediate delivery. If the woman is a Class A, B, or C diabetic, the doctor will probably check her estriol level weekly, or more often after her 30th week of pregnancy. If she's a Class D, F, or R diabetic, he'll check it daily 6 to 8 weeks before her expected due date.

Second, the doctor will monitor the baby's heart rate. A slowing heart rate indicates fetal distress and may mean it's time for immediate delivery.

If the estriol level and fetal heart rate stay stable in the third trimester, the doctor will perform an amniocentesis and check the L/S ratio about the 36th or 37th week. The L/S ratio will help him pinpoint the best time for delivery.

"What exactly is the L/S ratio?"

The L/S, or lecithin/sphingomyelin, ratio is an analysis of lung phospholipids in the amniotic fluid, which is an index of fetal lung maturity. One of the main dangers of delivering a baby prematurely is development of respiratory distress syndrome. When the L/S ratio reaches 1.8:1 to 2:1, the baby has much less chance of developing respiratory syndrome.

To test the L/S level, the doctor will obtain a sample of the amniotic fluid by aspirating it through the mother's abdomen.

"I get the impression I'll need a lot of medical attention during pregnancy. How often should I see my doctor?"

If a diabetic has reason to believe that she's pregnant, she should see her physician as soon as possible. He'll do a thorough examination, including routine laboratory work and a complete history of her diabetes, to determine what class diabetic she is. In most cases, an obstetrician and an internist will see her every 2 weeks for the first and second trimester and once a week for the third trimester. At each appointment, they'll check her weight, blood pressure, blood-sugar level, and urine and examine her for signs of hydramnios and edema. They'll also check the fundus of her eyes frequently. They'll evaluate her diabetic control and make any necessary changes in her diet or medication.

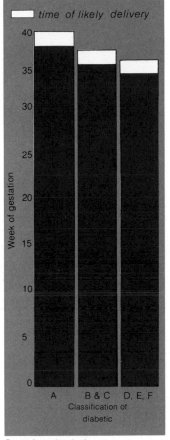

Carrying the baby
The more severe the mother's diabetes, the sooner physicians advise inducing labor to protect the health of mother and child.

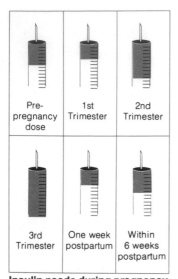

| Pre-pregnancy dose | 1st Trimester | 2nd Trimester |
| 3rd Trimester | One week postpartum | Within 6 weeks postpartum |

Insulin needs during pregnancy
During the first timester of pregnancy, insulin needs usually fall by one-third. In fact, hypoglycemic reactions can be the first indication of pregnancy.

In the second trimester insulin requirements rise to 66% above the prepregnancy dose, and by the last trimester the patient's need for insulin rises to twice the prepregnancy dosage.

For about five days or so after delivery, most mothers have a temporary remission in their diabetes. Their need for insulin drops dramatically, to about two-thirds their prepregnancy dose. But within six weeks they generally return to their normal insulin dosage.

Just before the birth of her baby, a diabetic should contact a pediatrician to be present during delivery. Most babies do well during delivery, but a pediatrician should be on hand to handle any problems that might arise.

"Will I be able to take oral hypoglycemic agents during pregnancy?"

Most authorities don't recommend it. Oral hypoglycemic agents may not adequately control hyperglycemia, which could harm the baby. Also, the sulfonylureas (tolbutamide, chlorpropamide, acetohexamide, and tolazamide) cross the placental barrier and enter the fetal circulation, which may cause prolonged hypoglycemia and possibly fetal death. If a woman is taking oral hypoglycemic agents before pregnancy, her doctor will probably switch her to insulin for the duration of her pregnancy.

"Will my insulin requirements change during pregnancy?"

Yes. In fact, they'll probably fluctuate. Insulin requirements frequently decrease during the first trimester. This effect isn't completely understood, but may be due to the utilization of glucose by the fetoplacental unit. Insulin requirements usually increase during the second and third trimesters, due to the insulin-antagonist state that results primarily from the placenta's production of hormones such as estrogen, progesterone, and lactogen as the placenta enlarges. It also results from a slight elevation in the free T_4 (thyroxine) and a slight increase in an adrenal cortical hormone known as cortisol. An insulin-degrading enzyme in the placenta, known as insulinase, also may increase the insulin requirement. At any rate, decreased insulin requirements during the second and third trimesters may indicate a failing placenta.

"What about my diet? Should I stick to it during pregnancy?"

Yes, but with a few slight changes to ensure that the mother and her baby get all the nutrients they need.

During pregnancy, a diabetic diet is modified to increase the carbohydrate intake. Severe restriction of carbohydrate could predispose a pregnant diabetic to ketosis, which could harm her baby. To supply the baby with enough glucose, she should take approximately 200 Gm of carbohydrate each day (800 calories). Total daily caloric requirement is 30 calories per kg of ideal body weight. If she's overweight, she may need to reduce her weight during pregnancy, but she shouldn't eat any less than 1400 calories per day.

A pregnant diabetic also should have a protein intake of about 1½ or 2 Gm per kg of ideal body weight. And she should keep fat intake stable.

Since excess weight will predispose her to toxemia, she should keep her weight gain to 15 pounds or less.

"Should I continue testing my urine for sugar and acetone?"
Yes. A pregnant diabetic should keep checking a second-voided specimen for sugar and acetone before meals and in the evening before bedtime. If urine sugar stays at 3+ or 4+ (1 to 2%) for more than three or four consecutive tests, she should report this to her doctor. If she gets a positive acetone reading, with or without sugar, she should report it to her doctor immediately. Acetone *without* sugar usually means that the woman isn't taking enough carbohydrates. Acetone *with* sugar often heralds the onset of ketoacidosis, which could cause fetal death in the second half of pregnancy.

During lactation, Benedict's and Clinitest urine sugar tests will be totally unreliable. That's because lactose, or milk sugar, spills into urine, giving high positive readings on these tests. During lactation, a diabetic can use Tes-Tape since it tests glucose specifically. Still, as a rapid testing method, it will indicate only a range of concentration rather than an absolute value. Remember that pregnancy creates a low renal threshold for glucose. So, relying on urinalysis alone is not enough. A pregnant diabetic also should have frequent blood sugar analyses.

"How would my insulin requirement be handled during delivery?"
Most likely the doctor will admit a pregnant diabetic to the hospital a few days before delivery to ensure maximum control of her diabetic state before and during delivery. On the day of delivery — either natural, induced, or cesarean section — he'll reduce her pregnancy dose of intermediate-acting insulin to half. After that, he'll tell you to keep her NPO on an intravenous infusion of 5% dextrose in water at a rate of 1000 cc every 8 hours until the woman has delivered and can eat normally.

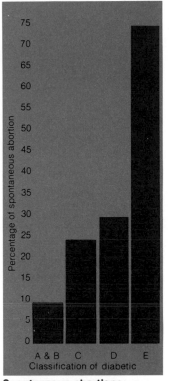

Spontaneous abortions
Expectant diabetics sometimes worry that their diabetes will prevent them from carrying their baby to term. Reassure them that the risk of spontaneous abortion is far smaller than it once was. Of course, the more severe an expectant mother's diabetes is, the greater a risk she runs in losing her child. In all but the most severe diabetics, though, chances of delivery far outweigh chance of spontaneous abortion.

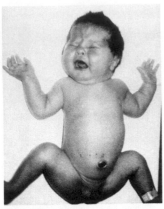

Norman Kendall, MD

A matter of size
This baby's mother is a diabetic; as a result at birth the baby weighed 9 lbs. 11 oz., large for her gestational age. Class A and B diabetics as well as mothers who develop diabetes during pregnancy often have heavy babies even though many are born prematurely. These babies lose the excess weight, largely due to fluid, shortly after birth.

The doctor will have blood sugars done every 4 to 6 hours and glucose elevations covered with Regular insulin every 4 to 6 hours as needed.

At the time of delivery, and usually for 48 to 72 hours afterwards, insulin requirements drop dramatically to the point where insulin may not be needed at all. During this period, the mother should be watched closely for signs of hypoglycemia. Her insulin requirements will return to the pre-pregnancy state within a week. If she has gestational diabetes, she may not need insulin after delivery after all.

"Will I be able to breast-feed my baby?"
Yes. The only caution is that a diabetic mother remain on insulin if she's been taking oral hypoglycemic agents prior to the pregnancy. Studies have confirmed that oral hypoglycemic agents get into the milk of lactating women. They haven't confirmed any adverse effect on nursing babies yet, but hypoglycemia in the infant is a possibility. To be on the safe side, a diabetic mother probably shouldn't take them if she's nursing her baby.

Because of nurses' expanding role, you have the good fortune to serve as patient counselor and instructor in diabetology, family planning, and prenatal and postnatal care. As an important member of the medical team, you can help ensure optimum success in diabetic pregnancies.

All the above answers will help you explain the truth and dispel the fictions about diabetic pregnancy. So, when a patient asks you, "Should I have a baby?" you can say, "I can't decide for you. But here are some facts that will help you better decide for yourself."

16

BLIND DIABETICS: BREEDING INDEPENDENCE

BY JOYCE SCHULZ, RN, AND
MARIE WILLIAMS, BA, MSW

WHY TRY TO make a blind diabetic independent? Isn't it easier just to make sure that his family, friends, or clinic will premeasure his insulin and test his urine? In fact, isn't it safer?

Yes, management by others is easier and maybe a little safer. And some blind diabetics may prefer it. But most blind diabetics, even those with supportive spouses, crave independence. And nearly all but the most severely diabetic could achieve it *if encouraged to*. Unfortunately, though, few health professionals give that encouragement. Too many of them feel that treatment should aim at absolute control with no risks. As well-meaning as that goal is, it overlooks the chief concern of many blind diabetics: a fulfilling life with minimal dependence on sighted persons. The health professionals' fears also reinforce those of the patient.

In our experience at the Minneapolis Society for the Blind, working primarily with diabetics, we've come to feel that you can't work adequately with a blind diabetic unless you understand the emotional impact of his blindness, its effect on diabetic control, and the practical skills that he can learn to control his condition. Sometimes it's necessary to de-emphasize diabetic control in favor of attention to the patient's emotional needs.

A double blow

Blindness comes as a tremendous shock to anyone, even an otherwise healthy person or someone whose vision has been fading for years. Suddenly the blind person realizes that he can't do all those things that we take for granted in everyday life — reading, writing, applying cosmetics, shaving, working, even just walking around freely. Since all of these activities are tied to our sense of self-worth, the most common reaction of any newly blind person is to feel that he's lost his worth as a person. He's still the person he was before, with all the same needs and goals. But to live a "normal" life, he has to start from scratch and relearn even the simplest activity.

Still, if blindness is a person's only handicap, he can usually master new techniques — traveling with a cane or dog, for instance; reading Braille; typing instead of writing; using special devices to cook, keep house, work.

For the diabetic, though, blindness comes as a double blow. Because of related health difficulties — loss of tactile sensitivity, for instance, or circulatory impairment — he may have more difficulty using Braille, moving around well, or keeping up with a job. Worst of all, blindness interferes with two activities essential to his very existence: Giving himself insulin injections and testing his urine. Still, the motivation of most blind diabetics is truly extraordinary; they want these skills so much that their desire often outweighs any difficulties.

Unfounded concerns about injections

Our experience indicates that, contrary to the assumption of some health professionals and patients, self-management of diabetes by blind patients needn't be dangerous or impossible. Of the more than 100 blind diabetics we've worked with, only a very few of those who wanted to become independent failed to learn how to measure and inject their insulin.

Many professionals and patients voice two concerns about self-injections: First, that the patient might inject a dangerous amount of air into subcutaneous tissue and, second, that he'll make a dangerous injection into a blood vessel. Let us lay both concerns to rest.

If a patient is taught proper techniques, he can't inject more than a harmlessly tiny amount of air into subcutaneous tissue. The only real danger to guard against is getting an air bubble so large that it displaces a significant quantity of insulin. By

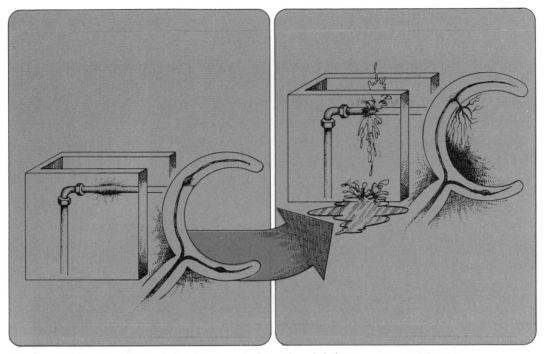

slowly withdrawing and reinjecting insulin into the vial three times before the actual injection and by holding the vial perpendicular to keep the insulin level, though, he can eliminate any large bubbles.

If the patient uses prescribed injection sites and techniques, he also runs little risk of injecting into a blood vessel — even though he won't be able to pull back the plunger to check for blood.

To make insulin injections as risk-free as possible, we also teach the following precautions:

• When giving himself an injection, the patient should stabilize his hand by placing his little finger against the skin and using it to locate the injection site. He then should inject the needle from the skin rather than with the more common dart-like motion. (Of course, there's no need to pull back on the plunger.)

• The patient must keep an accurate record of how many doses he's used so he'll know when his bottle is empty. One method of keeping an accurate record involves putting as many marbles as doses in a container and removing one marble after each injection. To keep the insulin level from getting too low, he should throw the bottle away when two doses remain.

Like a leaky pipe
In background retinopathy, blood vessel abnormalities are contained within the retina. The leakage from the vessels may be compared to a leaking pipe that damages plaster and wallpaper. In proliferative retinopathy, a more serious problem, blood vessels hemorrhage through the retina surface into the vitreous, like a pipe breaking through a wall and leaking water into a room.

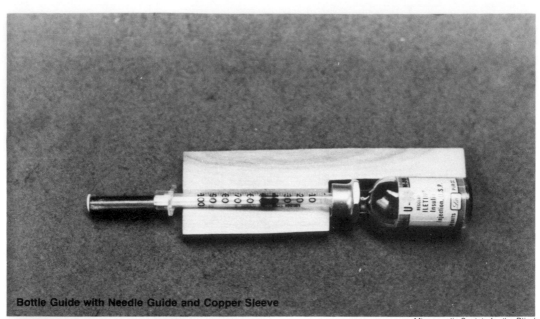

Bottle Guide with Needle Guide and Copper Sleeve

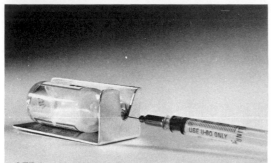

AFB Insulin Needle Guide

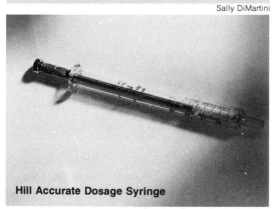

Hill Accurate Dosage Syringe

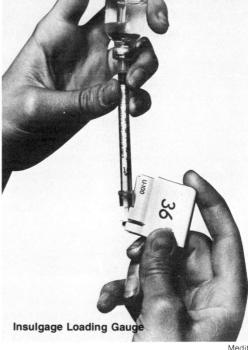

Insulgage Loading Gauge

Blind diabetics can use a variety of devices to measure their insulin accurately. We've found the Hill Accurate Dosage Syringe, the Copper Sleeve, and the Insulgage Loading Gauge useful and easy to manage. But you have to select each device to fit the particular patient's needs. Here are just some of the devices now available.

• *Hill Accurate Dosage Syringe.* Available through the American Foundation for the Blind and through some hospital supply companies, this reusable metal and glass syringe is readily obtainable for U-40 and U-80 insulin but more difficult to obtain for U-100. A sighted person has to pre-set the syringe, and the patient has to keep it sterile as he would any other reusable glass syringe. Only a doctor or nurse can order this device.

• *The Copper Sleeve.* This prototype for many loading devices is available through the Minneapolis Society for the Blind. The copper sleeve is a piece of copper tubing cut to the required dose with an individual glass or BD disposable syringe and fitted around the plunger. Usually patients find it simpler to use than the Hill Accurate Dosage Syringe, but some may find it too small to handle easily. The copper sleeve can't be used with different brands of syringes, to measure a mixed dose, or to vary a dose.

• *The Insulgage Loading Gauge.* This new device, manufactured by Meditec (Englewood, Colorado), is rapidly becoming the method of choice. It comes as a precalibrated volume regulator made of durable plastic and available in three dosage sizes — U-40, U-80, and U-100. Since insulin syringes may differ in size and shape, a gauge must be used exclusively with a particular brand and type. Currently gauges are available only for the disposable B D Plastipak self contained syringes and for Jelco long syringes. They come in sets of 2, 3, 5, 8, and 12, enabling the patient to vary his dosage or measure a mixed dose. They also come in standard ink print, raised numbers, or Braille.

In addition to these measuring devices, a blind diabetic may find the following useful.

• *Needle Guide.* Available from the American Foundation for the Blind, this small funnel-shaped metal device fits over the top of Eli Lilly insulin vials to help guide the needle into the rubber cap.

• *Bottle Guide.* Available from the Minneapolis Society for

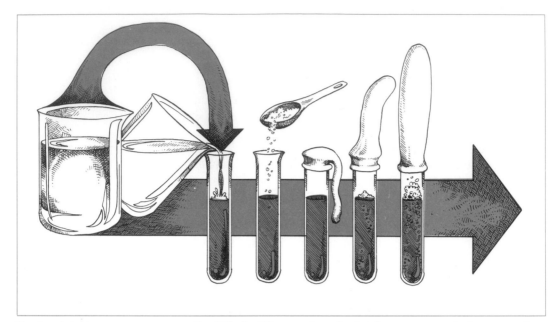

The touch test
Blind diabetics may test their urine themselves at home by adding yeast and testing the pressure of a fingercot with their hands. Although the method isn't foolproof, it can provide reassurance and a sense of independence for the patient.

the Blind, this wooden device has an extended arm against which the patient rests his bottle and a groove into which he places the syringe. He then slides the syringe along the groove and into the bottletop. Usually patients use this device along with the metal needle guide.

Urine testing: Not perfect, not essential
More than self-injections, self-testing of urine poses a problem to blind diabetics. Recently researchers developed a sound test for urine concentration. But so far all commonly available, reliable tests do depend on vision — a handicap to blind diabetics living alone.

We demonstrate the "yeast method" of urine testing to all of our blind diabetic patients. This method calls for placing ¼ teaspoon of yeast in a Uritec-tube and adding approximately 12 cc of urine. The patient then fits a fingercot over the top of the tube, making sure it is completely deflated. If glucose is present, it will interact with the yeast to form a gas that will inflate the fingercot within 10 to 20 minutes. By feeling the fingercot, the patient can assess the amount of glucose spillage: a deflated fingercot indicates no glucose or only a trace, a mushy feeling indicates a medium amount of glucose, and a taut feeling indicates a large amount of glucose.

Several of our blind patients use this method for reassurance on special occasions, such as when their spouse goes out of town for several days. But some diabetics refuse to use it because it's cumbersome, time-consuming, messy, and not totally reliable. We never condemn a patient who chooses not to use it. Naturally we always encourage urine testing. But we also accept the fact that not all patients will stick with it. And until someone invents a reliable, acceptable test that doesn't depend on vision, we feel we have no right to deny the blind diabetic the freedom to live independently without urine testing — provided he knows the risks.

Remember, most of the blind diabetics you work with will be familiar with the techniques of handling a syringe and giving themselves injections. If they want to become independent, most need nothing more than your reassurance to learn the simple modifications necessary to achieve it.

Your attitudes are critical, perhaps even paramount, in shaping the diabetic's state of mind and self-esteem when he first begins to lose vision. Long before a rehabilitation professional sees the person, you can facilitate his adaptation to life. The important thing is to focus not on what he has lost, but rather on the abilities he still has intact.

SKILLCHECK 4

1. Johnny Stover, 12-years-old, is on a 2600-calorie diet of three meals and three snacks. He also takes a split dose of insulin, one dose before breakfast and one before dinner. Three days a week, Johnny plays Little League baseball after school. What adjustments would you advise him to make on those days?

2. Several months ago, 2-year-old Mary Willis was discovered to have diabetes when she was brought into the hospital with convulsive hypoglycemic reactions. Since then, Mrs. Willis has been terrified of negative urine results. But she is trying to keep Mary on a strict routine that will keep her diabetes under complete control around the clock. How would you educate Mrs. Willis about Mary's diabetic condition?

3. Fifteen-year-old Terry is going through a trying adolescence. She is denying her diabetes and hiding it from her friends because "they wouldn't want to hang around with someone who's sick all the time." How could you help Terry develop a more positive outlook on her disease?

4. Debby Rosen developed diabetes at the age of 11. She is now 27 and wants to begin a family. However, she and her husband are concerned about pregnancy. Debby says she doesn't have any complications from her diabetes and she controls it well. But she's afraid pregnancy will make her diabetes worse. What would you tell her?

5. Ed Phillips is 44 years old. His visual acuity is: OD — counting fingers at 1 foot; OS — no light perception. Right now he is living with his brother, but in a few months he'll be living by himself in an apartment. Although he must move to be close to the radio station where he'll be working, Mr. Phillips is apprehensive about managing his diabetes alone. How would you prepare him for his move?

6. Eileen Shaunnessy, age 53, has managed her insulin injections well for nearly 10 years. Now, however, her sight is failing and she has trouble making sure she's drawing up the right amount of insulin and eliminating air bubbles. What would you recommend?

7. Nancy Byers, who controls her diabetes with 100 mg Tolinase daily, has just learned that she's pregnant with her first child. She's delighted but concerned about taking her Tolinase during pregnancy. She's heard it will hurt the baby and says she's going to stop taking it. What would you tell her?

8. Ted Nichols is 16 and on a daily dose of 8 units Regular insulin and 28 units NPH. He's planning to go backpacking in the Rockies. Although Ted has always been active, a backpacking trip will be slightly more active than he's used to. How would you advise him to plan for his trip?

9. Susan Hendricks has delivered a 9-pound, 4-ounce baby girl by Cesarean section. She has decided to breast-feed her baby, which means she will continue taking insulin rather than go back to her usual dose of DBI. On her first day home, Susan tests her urine with her Clinitest tablets and gets a reading of 3+. Very upset, she calls you and asks what to do. Should she take more insulin?

HOW TO GIVE IN-HOSPITAL CARE

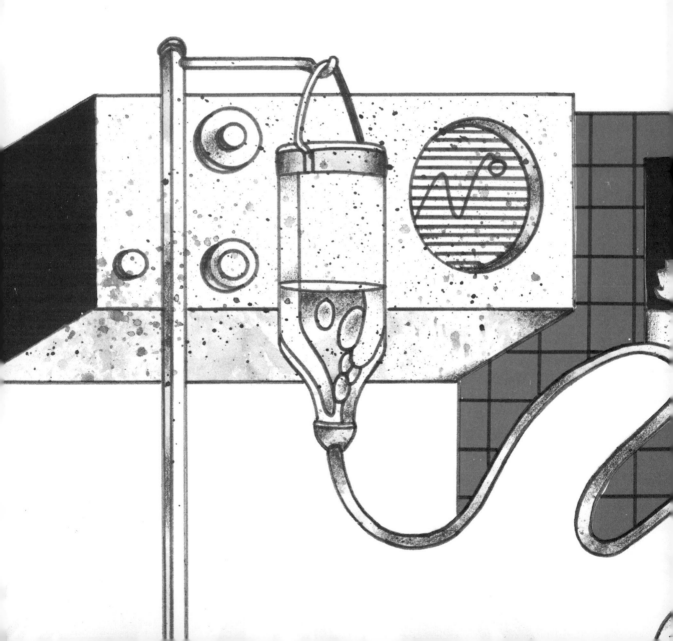

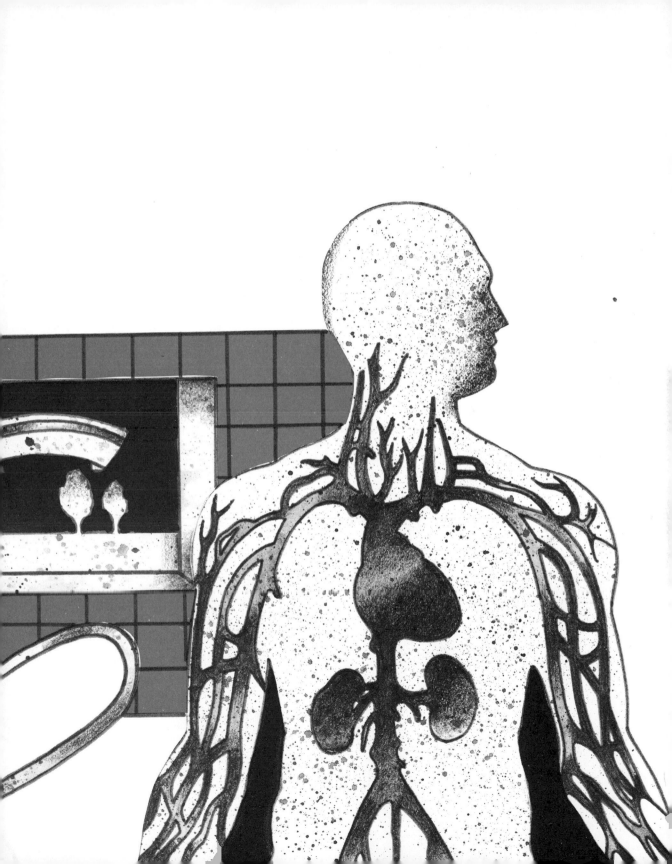

17
SKIRTING ILL EFFECTS OF SURGERY

BY EDWINA A. McCONNELL, RN, MS

SURGERY IS STRESS enough to the healthy patient: It challenges all the body's systems, including metabolism. For the diabetic patient, it looms larger still. With his own metabolism already more or less balanced on a seesaw, where keto-acidosis could await him if he slips off to one side and insulin shock if he tilts too far to the other, he faces a special situation. Not only do illness, surgery, and convalescence interrupt his normal food intake, his eating schedule and any insulin or medication program he may follow, but something else happens to intensify the effects of the interruption.

What happens is this.

His regimen has been aimed at controlling his blood glucose levels on an everyday plane, but now stress releases ACTH from the pituitary. The ACTH stimulates the adrenal cortex to produce glucocorticoids. These hormones increase gluconeogenesis — chemical breakdown of body fats and proteins into extra glucose — and the extra glucose goes directly into the bloodstream. Meantime, the catecholamine epinephrine, also normally released under stress to prepare the body for a fight or flight, spurs the conversion of stored glycogen to available glucose; this, too, raises the blood sugar. That calls for more insulin.

A typical case is Angela S., 23, a magazine staff writer who was hospitalized for a cystoscopy because of recurrent microscopic amounts of blood in her urine. Angela had been diagnosed as having diabetes a year earlier.

Since then, she had followed a diet based on 1,875 calories; 188 grams of it were carbohydrate, 94 protein, and 83 fat, a typical diabetic diet based on 15 calories to the pound of body weight with a ratio of 40-20-40% carbohydrate, protein, and fat, respectively. Angela's current insulin regimen was 20 units of Lente (or intermediate-acting) insulin and 10 units of Semilente (that is, short-acting) insulin daily before breakfast.

Her urine was normally sugar-free, or showed only a trace. Once or twice during regulation, she had reported preliminary symptoms of shock to her doctor. Yet the evening she was hospitalized, her urine showed 3+ sugar. But she gave no sign of an infection. We decided that the stress of anxiety was probably the culprit.

Angela S. was anxious about the next day's procedure and its possible revelation. She was quite worried about cancer, which ran in her family. All this anxiety was throwing her conscientiously regulated metabolism to the winds.

The problems of metabolic regulation we encountered with Angela are the essential ones faced by every diabetic patient undergoing surgery — and his doctor and his nurse. Such a patient needs a consistently stable internal environment. That means we need to:

— prevent severe fluid loss brought about through the osmotic diuresis forced by hyperglycemia;

— prevent ketosis that would follow insulin deficiency;

— prevent the diabetic coma that could follow ketoacidosis; *but also*

— ward off the opposite, hypoglycemia and insulin shock.

As a bonus, these steps also minimize the patient's predisposition to infection and spare his body any wasting of protein that he needs for tissue repair.

Just how you will do this depends, of course, on the doctor's preferences for treating diabetes. And it depends on other things such as the severity of the diabetes and its type of onset, as well as the presence of any diabetic complications. It also depends on any coexisting conditions and on the nature of the surgery.

As for severity and type, the patient with *mild* diabetes of mature onset (usually someone much older than Angela), is likely to be on a diet or diet-and-tablet regimen for control. He is usually able to tolerate the stress of either minor or major surgery with little metabolic disturbance — provided he has no infection. (Infection is one of the stresses that raises blood sugar.) He may be able to get through a minor procedure under a local anesthetic, in fact, with little change in his daily management.

The *moderate* diabetic is apt to be controlling his blood sugar by daily doses of intermediate-acting insulin, sometimes in conjunction with Regular (short-acting) insulin, as Angela's was controlled. The day of surgery he can usually be safely managed (if he has no infection) with intravenous glucose and a probaby reduced insulin dose, one cut by at least half.

The juvenile diabetic patient, generally in the ranks of those with *severe* diabetes, is apt to be classified as "brittle." His metabolic control during surgery is apt to be the most difficult.

Insulin needs can also swing wildly when an occasional patient develops insulin resistance. In this, thousands of units bind with insulin antibodies. However, most patients with this problem ultimately require large doses of insulin — usually greater than 200 units per day.

As for the nature of surgery, the terms "minor" and "major" denote the total stresses associated with a surgical procedure. This not only means the extent of physical trauma involved (including that of organ manipulation and the amount of tissue incised and sutured), but also the length of time the operation takes, the anesthetic agent used, and — underlying it all, of course — the patient's psychological response. Major surgical procedures lasting several hours, such as radical mastectomy, thoracotomy, subtotal gastrectomy, or abdominal perineal resection, cause the greatest disruption in metabolic control. Minor procedures such as cystoscopy, cataract removal, dilatation and curettage, and tooth extractions cause the least. Certainly a cystoscopy was not exactly a major procedure — except to Angela S., and to anyone who could understand why she might be concerned.

Individualizing nursing care

Each patient is a unique human being with individual needs and ways of coping. The patient undergoing surgery, with or without diabetes, is indisputably no exception. Major or minor

Common diabetic conditions
No pathological difference exists between the surgical conditions of diabetics and those of normal patients. But diabetics are more prone to several conditions that may require surgery. Among them: gallstones, cancer of the pancreas and general malignant disease, Dupuytren's contracture, soft tissue infection, and gangrene of the extremities.

to you, the surgery will be major to him. Not only is his body the target of a planned assault, but his mind becomes a breeding ground for anxiety, conjecture, and concern. If you can work with the patient preoperatively, that may relieve some of his anxiety and facilitate a smoother postoperative course. Assess each patient, and, together with him, plan his care.

Preoperatively he will probably need the following lab tests and studies:
— fasting blood sugar
— postprandial blood sugar
— routine urine with emphasis on sugar and acetone
— CBC
— BUN
— serum electrolytes
— EKG
— chest films.

And he should have a blood sugar drawn 1 hour preoperatively. If the level turns out to be low, he's going to need a glucose infusion (D_5W) to keep from becoming hypoglycemic during surgery. But, regardless of the blood sugar results, *all* insulin dependent diabetic patients should have an intravenous access throughout surgery should any problems arise. Angela's urine sugar had been brought down to 1+ with 10 units of Regular insulin just before surgery. Her doctors were satisfied to have a slight margin of reserve sugar on hand to ward off hypoglycemia, which can be dangerous and hard to detect in an unconscious patient.

For the usual diabetic patient, the dosage of preop morphine or meperidine will be reduced by one quarter or one half. Why? The nausea and vomiting that these drugs can all too easily cause will *decrease* his need for insulin, enhancing his chances of a hypoglycemic reaction. (Nausea and vomiting have an effect quite opposite that of infection or fever which, like stress, is known to raise the blood sugar.)

Understanding methods of control
Physicians use numerous methods to keep the patient free of ketoacidosis and acetonuria, dehydration, and hypoglycemia and its shock. You must be familiar with the methods used, and be acutely aware of the treatment course chosen for *your* patient. Here are several of the methods most commonly used by specialists.

Mild diabetes. If the patient usually takes an oral hypoglycemic agent and can do so the day of surgery, this method should be continued. Each missed meal can be replaced with 50 grams of intravenous glucose.

But if the patient can't tolerate oral medication, a dose of subcutaneous insulin would be given the morning of surgery, with missed meals being made up by the glucose. Remember, though, unless he can eat to make up for it, a patient who takes the oral agent chlorpropamide (Diabinese) shouldn't be given any insulin for 36 hours, because that's the half-life of the drug.

Moderate diabetes. For the patient whose diabetes is daily controlled by intermediate-acting insulin, alone or combined with Regular (short-acting) insulin, I.V. infusions of D_5W or $D_{10}W$ will provide the necessary carbohydrates. Once the infusion has been started, a reduced dose of the usual insulin mixture, from one-third to one-half the normal maintenance dose, is given subcutaneously.

The reduced dose will avoid the very serious threat of insulin shock on the operating table.

Specialists feel that transient hyperglycemia would be far less harmful. But in this method, closer postoperative observation is needed against elevated blood sugar. In fact, some specialists recommend giving the withheld part of the insulin dose when the patient reaches the recovery room after taking a STAT blood sugar and evaluating the patient's needs.

But if infection is present, either the mild or the moderate diabetic will probably need to be treated like a severe diabetic.

Severe diabetes. Here is one preferred method for treating the patient with severe diabetes, or the patient with lesser diabetes but with a fever or infection: Assess the patient's metabolic status every 1 to 6 hours. The daily CHO requirements, given as a 5 or 10% glucose either in water or in an electrolyte solution, are divided into 6-hour infusions. With the beginning of each 6-hour infusion, Regular insulin is given, subcutaneously. The slow infusion is continued through and after surgery until the patient can eat again, and both its glucose content and the insulin given are determined by the serum glucose.

For most patients, Regular insulin is usually given by 5-unit increments for every 1 + sugar on the reagent scale. That is, for a 4+ Clinitest reaction, 15 units of Regular insulin should ordinarily bring the blood sugar down to 1+. If there is

Postop mortality is declining
Thanks to Banting's discovery of insulin in 1920 the postop mortality rate for diabetics fell dramatically in the 20s and 30s. Recent medical advances have cut the mortality rate even further. For example, in 3551 operations on diabetic patients at the New England Deaconess Hospital during the first eighteen years (1923-41) after the discovery of insulin, the mortality rate was 7.3. In the 19 years between 1950 and 1969 operations totaled 9484 and the mortality rate had dropped to 2.65.

acidosis, another 5 units may be given.

Ketoacidosis is a critical problem that must be managed by carefully evaluating blood sugar levels, electrolytes and pH as well as the patient's clinical status.

The following five methods of control are also often used.

1. Some physicians withhold glucose and insulin until the postoperative period instead of using the method outlined above. This does prevent hypoglycemia during surgery, but it increases the possibility of postoperative diabetic keto-acidosis.

2. Another method of control divides equally the daily car-bohydrate and insulin doses. The carbohydrate is given paren-terally in four periods, usually every 6 hours. Regular insulin in doses one-fourth the size of the usual total daily requirement is given subcutaneously. Urine specimens are used to ascertain the dosage of supplemental insulin needed.

To determine that dosage, fractional urines for sugar and acetone are used — all the urine passed at a specific period throughout the day, most often before meals and at bedtime. But a word of caution: don't collect urine that's been sitting in the patient's bladder overnight or even for several hours, because it will tell more about the past than about the present so far as spilling sugar or acetone into the urine is concerned. Instead, test the second voided specimen.

To obtain a urine specimen from a patient with a Foley catheter, simply clamp the catheter for 15 to 30 minutes. Then, clean the catheter with an alcohol wipe and aspirate a small amount of urine using a 25 gauge needle to puncture the catheter. *Do not disconnect* the catheter from its tubing. This would give microorganisms easy access to the bladder of someone who is most vulnerable to infection.

But before testing the urine for sugar and acetone, note what medications the patient is getting. With Clinitest tablets, large quantities of ascorbic acid, NegGram, the cephalosporins, or probenecid can give false-positive readings. Yet, except for ascorbic acid, these medications have no effect on glucose testing done with Tes-Tape, Hema-Combistix, Combistix, Uristix, Clinistix, Keto-Diastix, or Diastix.

3. The next method of control for the severe diabetic patient during surgery is the one described earlier as satisfactory for the moderate diabetic. It uses insulin preoperatively in re-duced doses, followed by postoperative supplements. Fre-

HOW TO CARE FOR A SURGICAL DIABETIC ADEQUATELY CONTROLLED WITH DIET AND NPH OR LENTE INSULIN

Before surgery
- Don't make any change in insulin or diet regimen.

Day of the operation

In early morning
- Omit breakfast.
- Start I.V. infusion of 1,000 ml 10% glucose in water or saline solution, to be infused over 6-8 hours.
- Give approximately half of the patient's usual daily dose of insulin subcutaneously when you begin the glucose infusion.

On completion of operation
- Give remaining half of the patient's usual daily dose of NPH or Lente insulin subcutaneously.
- Continue I.V. infusion of 5 or 10% glucose in water or saline solution (generally ¼-⅓ of total fluid should be saline solution) so that the patient receives a total of approximately 200 Gm of glucose in 2,000-3,000 ml of fluids in the first 24 hours. You may need to modify this depending on the patient's fluid and electrolyte needs. Just make sure you give at least 200 Gm glucose daily.
- Give oral fluids and food as soon as patient's condition permits.
- Check urine sugar and ketones every 4 hours postoperatively (if patient can void) and blood glucose and plasma ketones every 4-6 hours. Obtain the first determinations as soon as the patient returns from the operation. Don't try to keep strict control of hyperglycemia or glucosuria. If the patient has moderate or severe ketonuria, serum ketones become elevated, or the blood sugar exceeds 250-300 mg/100 ml, give 5-20 units of Regular insulin subcutaneously.

Days following the operation
- Give the patient his usual dose of NPH or Lente insulin. If he is to be maintained entirely on continuous I.V. fluids for several days, give the insulin as two equal doses 12 hours apart.
- Resume usual preoperative diet or a diet comparable in calories as soon as postoperative condition permits.
- If patient can't be fed orally or oral intake is inadequate, give I.V. infusion of 5 or 10% dextrose in water to total approximately 200 Gm carbohydrate/24 hours until the patient's condition permits return to his usual diet.

quent testing of the urine for sugar may be needed.

4. A fourth method adjusts diabetic management to the patient, the surgical procedure, and the disease for which the surgery is performed. Insulin of the usual type is given in the usual dose at the regular time. Each missed meal is replaced with 50 grams of I.V. glucose.

Because his stomach is empty, the patient can go to surgery at any time, and the I.V. glucose feedings are used to offset the daily insulin until he can tolerate oral feedings once again. Supplemental requirements of Regular insulin in addition to this regimen are determined by the patient's clinical condition and the degree and persistence of glycosuria and any ketonuria. But if there *is* ketonuria, be sure not to classify it strictly as a sign of impending diabetic ketoacidosis. Think also of infection and even of dehydration or starvation.

5. And then some physicians like to infuse Regular insulin along with the intravenous glucose. Depending on the vessel used to hold it, insulin is usually stable and does not stratify in either 5 or 10% solutions of dextrose and water, with or

without electrolytes. But there are enough other variables in this method to have caused its replacement in many centers. Simultaneous infusion of both glucose solution and insulin should afford smoother control of the diabetes, true? Yet, in fact, it gives poor dosage control and can produce fluctuations of the blood glucose level. This is because, when insulin is administered in I.V. solutions, a large percentage of it may adhere to both the bottle and the tubing, sending through a greatly reduced dose. Then if the same tubing were to be used for more than one infusion, insulin by now might have saturated the binding sites on the tube walls so that the comparative increase in free circulating insulin could precipitate a hypoglycemic reaction. Another variable: If the I.V. solutions are changed halfway through the bottle — say, D_5W is replaced with D_5W/lactates — the real dosage is once more unpredictable.

If you *must* add insulin to the I.V., be sure it's Regular insulin to avoid delayed reactions. And be sure to change the tubing, preferably with every bottle, but at least every 24 hours.

Goals of postoperative care

Again, the primary goal is the patient's stability. This means reestablishing control of the diabetes, looking after the patient's emotional well-being, preventing infection, and promoting the healing of the surgical wound.

Usually, because the stress of surgery is diminished postoperatively, the insulin requirements also decrease — especially if a source of infection was removed. But if the patient is still stressed and anxious, and particularly if the surgery has altered his body image or confirmed a diagnosis that could change his life-style, they will hardly be lower, and they might even rise. Each individual's coping mechanisms are different.

Your nursing care of the patient will include:
— checking and evaluating the vital signs
— measuring intake and output
— checking dressings for drainage
— monitoring all tubes for patency and function
— conscientiously observing I.V. infusions
— accurately recording all the above data
— taking fractional urines if ordered.
Besides these things, you must observe your patient carefully

for signs of either impending diabetic ketoacidosis (coming from too little insulin) or hypoglycemia (coming from too much).

DKA not only may come from insufficient natural insulin or an inadequate or omitted insulin dosage, but also from acute illness or medications that similarly raise the blood sugar, such as cortisone. Since the metabolic derangement here is hyperglycemia, the treatment is insulin.

Hypoglycemia or insulin shock results not only from too much insulin, but also from omission or delay of meals; too much exercise without supportive food intake; or nutritional and fluid imbalances from nausea and vomiting. This, too, can turn into coma.

But up to a certain point, hypoglycemic shock is the more dangerous of the two. If severe enough, or if habitual, it can leave the patient who survives it with brain damage expressed as loss of memory, diminished ability to learn, or even paralysis. The central nervous system is acutely sensitive to glucose deprivation. When the blood sugar is high, as in ketoacidosis, the brain can still use available glucose even in the absence of insulin. But when the blood sugar is low, the brain is altogether robbed of the glucose it must have. Many physicians consider consistently spilling a little sugar into the urine preferable to too narrow a line of control with its risk of hypoglycemia.

On the afternoon of Angela S.'s cystoscopic examination, when she had been returned to her room, the nurse noticed that she seemed more than ordinarily sleepy for a patient out of anesthesia for several hours. She put her hand on the patient's forehead, then, and asked her how she felt. She received a rather drunken-sounding reply, and felt perspiration on Angela's forehead. She managed to arouse Angela enough to get her to take 4 ounces of orange juice, and then sent for a resident.

It turned out that the extra Regular insulin given that morning to control her hypoglycemia had thrown her into a slight reaction. Although the orange juice did offset it, a closer watch was kept. And a bottled sweet drink was set near the bed to be handy.

The treatment for insulin shock is sugar, given quickly. If your patient is awake, give 4 ounces of orange juice, two sugar lumps, or two teaspoons of honey as a starting dose — 10

Watch out for infections
Infections (especially staphylococcal and mixed gram-negative) are a grave problem among diabetics. During and after surgery the patient may undergo derangements of nervous system function so that he loses sensation in infected areas. Remember that you can't count on pain to warn you about infection, so watch closely for minor lesions that could become serious problems if unattended.

grams of CHO altogether. Sometimes, you'll need to start I.V. glucose even with patients who are still awake. The treatment for those already in coma is usually 20-50 ml of 50% intravenous glucose given by push. For those patients not in shock so long that their available liver glycogen stores have been exhausted, glucagon may be ordered.

When the insulin-shock patient recovers, the cause needs finding. It may mean reassessing his program.

These are the two sides of diabetes, then, two extreme derangements leading to coma and ultimate death if untreated, and two opposite treatments. Yet superficially, the two derangements may resemble each other. What of the confusion? Remember, whereas glucose given to a DKA patient even in coma need not spell the difference between life and death that minute, *insulin can kill a shock patient.*

Whenever there is a question between insulin hypoglycemia (shock) and diabetic ketoacidosis, always give the patient *sugar.* If it turns out to be DKA, little harm will have been done. If it is insulin shock, you will probably have saved a life!

Pending lab tests, what is the best way to check these patients for either threat? When the patient is sleeping, check for warm, dry skin and smell his breath for a *sweet, fruity odor* — that would be DKA. It is often accompanied by fast, *labored breathing* — a respiratory compensation for the metabolic acidosis.

Check for *diaphoresis* by touching his gown and pillow case; dampness would mean hypoglycemia. This may also be accompanied by nightmares or sleepwalking. If you wonder whether the patient is actually asleep or progressing quietly into coma, don't hesitate to awaken him.

And other nursing measures are special to the patient with diabetes mellitus. His susceptibility to infection, for example, means you should encourage him to cough and breathe deeply in order to minimize the possibility of pneumonia. Use scrupulous asepsis when catheterizing such a patient, caring for the catheters, or changing his dressing.

Premature peripheral vascular disease is another threat to the diabetic patient. Be doubly alert to any signs and symptoms of developing thrombophlebitis. Encourage the patient to turn and move to prevent decubiti, and to exercise his legs to prevent pulmonary emboli. Elastic support hose also help prevent thrombophlebitis. They should be removed every 8

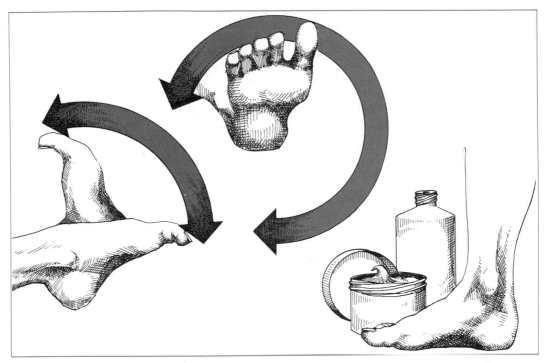

hours and the skin examined for redness and pressure sores. Keep his skin clean and dry, and *never* use ordinary adhesive tape on it.

Further management of the metabolism. Oral calorie intake is practically always preferable to intravenous feedings in a diabetic patient. As soon as possible after surgery, feed him and record the calories consumed. A progression to his usual diabetic diet will get him back on his normal regulated insulin dosage.

For the diabetic patient with nasogastric suction, postop or preop, be on your guard against acidosis, electrolyte imbalance, and dehydration. Carefully record the amounts of I.V. solutions given so as to calibrate the glucose calories the patient receives.

For the patient on hyperalimentation, Regular insulin is usually calculated and given to fit each patient's need. This need is determined by blood-sugar levels — for example, those over 200 mg/100 ml; by urine tests for sugar; and by the total calories being administered. If the hyperalimentated or, indeed, any diabetic patient spills 3+ sugar or more, look for sepsis that might be causing the hyperglycemia. Check cultures of urine and blood. Examine the area where the tubing is

Exercise even when ill
Bedridden diabetics must exercise to help circulation in their legs. They should extend and flex, abduct and adduct each foot ten times a day. If feet are dry, they should apply lanolin or cocoa butter to prevent cracking and lesions.

inserted and the tubing itself. Check the clinical signs and the patient's general well-being. The glucosuria should be covered with Regular insulin.

Be sure that your diabetic surgical patient is adequately hydrated. If he is protected against hypoglycemic shock by continuous mild hyperglycemia, then polyuria and gradual dehydration are a chronic threat. If they continue unchecked over a period, this could add up to another metabolic crisis: Hyperglycemic hyperosmolar nonketotic coma (HHNK). Treatment, rather than depending on insulin, stresses the replacement of the vast quantities of liquid wasted by the osmotic diuresis.

Teaching. Even though the patient may have had diabetes mellitus for several years, there will be gaps in his understanding of it and perhaps room for improvement in his carrying out his own regimen. Teach your diabetic patient whatever you can, and teach his family, too. A dietary consult well in advance of discharge may be helpful. Document your teaching plan.

When he is ready to leave, you may want to refer him to a community health agency or to some community health personnel. The doctor will decide what his regimen is, but your place in helping him understand it and carry it out can be critical.

18

GETTING READY FOR MEDICAL TESTS

BY CATHERINE GAROFANO, RN, BS

GIVEN THE SERIOUS NATURE of major surgery and illnesses and the changeable nature of diabetes, you'd expect a very ill or surgical diabetic to challenge all your nursing skills. The last chapter certainly confirmed your expectations.

But what would you expect with a diabetic undergoing a simple diagnostic procedure, such as a gastric analysis or an upper G.I. series? True, the nursing protocol may not be as intricate. But it's every bit as important as the protocol for a surgical diabetic. Because just a simple slip-up in your preparation or instructions can send the patient headlong into hypoglycemia or hyperglycemia and even ketoacidosis.

Consider, for example, Calvin Brown, an inpatient who was sent to the lab for a routine gastric analysis. Because he was scheduled for his test at 10 a.m. and was to be NPO beforehand, the floor nurse assumed she should withhold his usual insulin dose. The lab was backed up with patients, so Calvin waited...and waited. After 1½ hours, he began to feel tired, weak, and thirsty. When he began complaining of stomach cramps, the lab technicians called his floor. Fortunately the head nurse recognized the symptoms as hyperglycemia with possible ketoacidosis and ordered Calvin returned to the unit without delay. She contacted the doctor for orders to treat the hyperglycemia. Then she talked to Calvin's floor nurse and explained that because Calvin's appointment was so late in the morning, she should have asked the doctor about giving him part of his insulin and a slow drip of I.V. glucose to maintain blood-sugar control before and during the test. Or better yet, she should have had the test rescheduled for 7 a.m. so Calvin could stick to his normal routine.

Adhering to such simple guidelines will help you keep patients like Calvin Brown poised in diabetic balance before and after diagnostic tests. Here's a brief review.

No matter what

An insulin-dependent patient requires his insulin whether he eats or not. If he hasn't eaten, though, the dosage should be adjusted—to account not only for the lack of food but also for his hormonal milieu. As you'll remember from the last chapter, stressful situations, such as diagnostic tests, stimulate the production of certain hormones such as cortisol and epinephrine. These insulin antagonists in turn increase the body's insulin needs. So insulin dosages must be carefully calculated.

If at all possible, procedures for insulin-dependent diabetics should be performed first thing in the morning. That way, the patient will be able to take food and his usual insulin dose in the morning after he returns from the test.

With radiological procedures (such as a G.I. series, barium enema, or intravenous pyelogram) your hospital may have you give the patient only clear liquids or a simple carbohydrate diet the evening before the test. In planning for this meal and a bedtime snack, take care to check the caloric needs of a patient on an intermediate-acting insulin and to order foods that will cover them adequately.

The doctor must adjust the evening dose of insulin for patients who normally receive insulin both in the morning and in the evening. Be sure to watch these patients carefully through the night for signs of possible reactions—either hypoglycemia or hyperglycemia. Test their urine for sugar every 4 to 6 hours; give a liquid sugar, such as orange juice, or an injection of glucose or glucagon followed by an I.V. of dextrose to counteract hypoglycemia, and a small dose of Regular insulin as ordered by the doctor to counteract hyperglycemia.

The patient should be kept NPO the morning of the procedure. Some hospitals suggest that you withhold the morning dose of insulin until the patient has returned from the procedure and can eat. If this is standard in your hospital and the patient will probably miss one meal that day, reduce his insulin dose. A better approach when possible, though, is to give the patient half of his usual morning dose at the usual time and start him on an I.V. drip of 5% dextrose at the rate of 1000 ml per 8 hours. Continue the I.V. through the procedure. Afterwards, discontinue the I.V. Give the patient a small morning meal and the remainder of his insulin dose.

A minor reminder

As mentioned briefly in the last chapter, you usually don't have to specially prepare diabetics for minor surgical procedures performed under local anesthesia (such as dental extractions, removal of warts, and so on). But remember that these patients are more prone to infections than the average patient. So, some physicians will have you start a diabetic on prophylactic antibiotic therapy before or at the beginning of the procedure. Because these procedures generally produce little stress, the patient usually won't need to adjust his insulin dose. But check his urine sugar closely for a day or two after the procedure.

These precautions will keep your diabetic patient on an even keel throughout most any test—ready to return to his normal activities.

SKILLCHECK 5

1. Elliot Martin, 52 years old and an insulin-dependent diabetic, has gone into the hospital for excision of a benign tumor. Even though he knows the tumor is benign and the surgery is minor, Mr. Martin seems very nervous about the operation. He hasn't been eating well so he tells you to decrease his insulin dose. What would you tell him?

2. Francine Wilkes and Robert Upshaw, both diabetics, are on your medical-surgical unit awaiting surgery. A nursing student asks if you have a standard set of nursing rules for diabetic surgical patients. You tell her that care for diabetic patients has to be individualized. What five criteria would you use to individualize care for diabetics?

3. Michael MacDonnald, who controls his diabetes with Tolinase, is having outpatient diagnostic tests. He was scheduled for a 7 a.m. barium enema X-ray but, as usual, the radiology department is running behind schedule. Now, at 11:30 you find him in the hall still waiting for his X-ray. He seems very distracted, irritable, and shaky. What would you suspect?

4. Saul Jaffe, a diabetic usually controlled on oral agents, has been comatose from a stroke for 36 hours. Why must you test his urine for sugar and acetone every 1 to 6 hours? How would you take a urine specimen? What precautions should you observe when reading the results?

5. Ron Kominsky, who normally takes 26 units of NPH insulin every morning, is scheduled for a prostatectomy at 7:00 this morning. You're in charge of preparing him for surgery. What orders would the doctor give you?

6. Adele Wister, age 54, controls her diabetes with 500 mg Dymelor every morning. She is in the hospital now for a hysterectomy. To control her diabetes during hospitalization,

the doctor has switched her to 8 units of Regular insulin twice a day. After surgery, you check her urine every 6 hours for sugar and acetone. In her latest urine test, you find that she is spilling acetone. She is sweating profusely and sleeping fitfully. When you try to rouse her, she doesn't respond. What should you do?

SKILLCHECK ANSWERS

ANSWERS TO SKILLCHECK 1

Situation 1 — Morton O'Reilly
No. During his hospitalization, Mr. O'Reilly has been unusually sedentary, eating a special diet, and under a great deal of stress. All of these conditions could skew his GTT results. He should have a GTT at one of his follow-up visits in a month or two. (Several fasting or 2-hour postprandial glucose tests might be better than a GTT in some cases. However, a GTT is more convenient for the patient since it doesn't require multiple visits for lab work.)

Situation 2 — Willard Jones
No. Glucose values rise with age. Mr. Jones' glucose tolerance test would almost certainly be abnormal if interpreted by conventional criteria designed for generally healthy young adults; norms for elderly people aren't available. Instead of a GTT, Mr. Jones might have a 2-hour postprandial glucose determination. (Results below 225 mg/dl would be normal; results above 225 mg/dl could indicate a need for therapy, probably dietary adjustments.)

Situation 3 — Martha Simon
You could suggest two alternatives and let Ms. Simon take her pick. On her active days, she could eat a mid-morning snack of a slow-acting carbohydrate (crackers or bread) and a 9:00 or 9:30 snack of protein or fat. If her weight is normal and she has no trouble maintaining it, she would probably choose this alternative since her activity would burn off the additional calories. If Ms. Simon is overweight and is struggling to lose pounds, however, she might prefer to decrease her insulin dose on active days. To determine a realistic dose of insulin for active days, have her check her urine before lunch on those days.

Situation 4 — Julie
One piece of fruit, which is a fast-acting carbohydrate, usually won't control an insulin-dependent diabetic's glucose level for long. Julie should have a slower-acting carbohydrate with protein or fat to better control her nocturnal glucose levels. You might suggest crackers and cheese. If Julie doesn't want to increase her caloric intake, you could suggest that she decrease her dinner by a bread and meat exchange and then eat these later as a bedtime snack. Reducing her intake at dinner will improve her bedtime Clinitest results, and eating a bedtime snack will maintain her glucose levels throughout the night.

Situation 5 — Paul
Extreme hunger often signals elevated blood sugar levels. Paul appears to be caught on the treadmill of eating more food, leading to a higher blood sugar level, leading to increased urinary loss of glucose, leading to more hunger, leading to more eating. His rapid growth during adolescence also may have altered his insulin needs. To ensure Paul's full growth potential during adolescence, you must stabilize his diabetes. Paul may need to be hospitalized briefly to establish dietary control. Then, you can help Paul realistically evaluate his total caloric intake. Paul may not fit into the standard dietary guidelines and may find a high-calorie diet with substantial snacks better suited to his life-style and needs.

Situation 6 — Harold Jefferson
Mr. Jefferson is a poor candidate for oral hypoglycemic agents for two reasons. First, he is taking hydrochlorothiazide, a thiazide diuretic that may provoke hyperglycemia. In fact, he might find that his blood sugar levels would fall considerably if he switched to a different diuretic. Second, he also has cardiac problems; some studies have shown that oral agents, particularly the sulfonylureas, increase the risk of death from cardiac disease. Still, Harold could use oral agents if he were changed to another type of diuretic that wouldn't affect his blood sugar and if his doctor felt that oral therapy were best for Mr. Jefferson depite his cardiac problems. If Harold were to use oral agents, he could use only phenformin — not one of the sulfonylureas. Allergy to one sulfa drug often indicates allergy to all sulfa and sulfa-like drugs. Since Harold is allergic to sulfisoxazole, a sulfa derivative, chances are he'd be allergic to sulfonylureas, which are chemically related to sulfonamide antimicrobial drugs.

Situation 7 — Jane Scarlotti
The "funny taste" that Mrs. Scarlotti describes indicates that she's reached the maximum dose of phenformin that she can tolerate. The doctor should reduce her dose slightly. Since Mrs. Scarlotti's urine tests have been 0 to 1+, she seems to be maintaining good control. A slight reduction in dosage shouldn't affect her control, but it will eliminate the metallic taste. You should remind Mrs. Scarlotti that breath mints contain a lot of sugar, so she shouldn't use them. If she needs breath mints to cover the metallic taste until it disappears permanently, she should use the sugarless type.

Situation 8 — Sarah Steinman

There are several likely reasons for Ms. Steinman's variable response to insulin. She may be alternating the order of her insulins when she draws them up, causing variations in the mixture because of dead space. To ensure a constant response, she should draw up the insulins in the same order every day. Or, if she has periodic local reactions to injections, such as edema, absorption of the insulin may be delayed. This could account for the hypoglycemic reaction if she isn't getting food at the right time to counteract the insulin's initial impact. Or, Ms. Steinman may not be adjusting her insulin dose to coincide with variations in her level of activity or stress. Finally, she may have used contaminated or deteriorated insulin. Remind her to discard any "suspicious" insulin.

Situation 9 — Frank Fisher

You should explain to the student that oral hypoglycemic therapy is always a risk in hospitalized patients. The stress of hospitalization plus dietary changes in the hospital often cause diabetes to fluctuate considerably. Oral hypoglycemic agents can't control diabetes under these conditions. So, the patient should be switched to insulin during his hospital stay.

Mr. Fisher also has another problem that precludes oral therapy: congestive heart failure. Congestive heart failure predisposes him to lactic acidosis. Since phenformin also *may* predispose a patient to lactic acidosis, he'd be in double jeopardy. Insulin would definitely be the best therapy for him.

Situation 10 — Jacqueline Bond

If Ms. Bond will be eating a large lunch on some days, she should eat something on other days to establish consistency. She can obtain her carbohydrates, proteins, and fats in a quick meal, such as a hamburger, fruit, and perhaps potato chips or french fries. She should have her lunch calculated as both a full-course meal and as a quick meal. As for the cocktails at business lunches, Ms. Bond can accommodate the alcohol by lowering her fat consumption at lunch. Once Ms. Bond establishes a consistent diet, she may need to adjust her insulin to account for the changes in her eating habits.

ANSWERS TO SKILLCHECK 2

Situation 1 — Frank Melton

The elevation in Mr. Melton's urine sugar after supper and throughout the night may be caused simply by poor dietary habits. He may be eating an excessively large dinner or bedtime snack, which his insulin can't accommodate. If dietary control doesn't correct the problem, though, Mr. Melton could add an inter-mediate or long-acting insulin to his morning dose of insulin. That would give him better 24-hour control. If that doesn't work, though, he could take a small dose of intermediate insulin before dinner to guarantee overnight control.

Situation 2 — Gretchen Hanson

There are two potential errors in Gretchen's technique. First, she says she "shakes" the bottle. If that's true, she may be creating air bubbles or foam in the bottle, which would prevent her from drawing up an accurate dosage. You should remind her that she should mix the insulin *gently* by inverting the bottle a few times. Second, Gretchen doesn't say that she checks the syringe for air bubbles or tries to eliminate them. Remind her to look for them and to remove them by pulling the plunger back and then pushing it in to the correct number of units, by flicking the barrel of the syringe with her finger, or by pushing the insulin back into the bottle and drawing up another dose.

Of course, Gretchen also may be slipping off her diet or simply need a change in dosage.

One more error in Gretchen's technique bears mentioning, even though it wouldn't affect her dosage: She doesn't say that she washed her hands before starting an injection. Remind her how important this step is, since diabetics are susceptible to infections.

Situation 3 — Bill Preston

Mr. Preston will be on the plane about 8 hours, so he should take along a snack of crackers in case he experiences a hypoglycemic reaction. Since less than 24 hours will elapse between his insulin injection at home and his next injection in Paris, he probably should take a much smaller dose of Regular insulin and a somewhat smaller dose of NPH in Paris; his doctor can tell him exactly how much less to take. On subsequent mornings in Paris, he will take his usual dose. When returning, since less than 24 hours will elapse again, he should follow the same protocol he followed on the trip over.

Situation 4 — Jill Collins

First, tell Jill that she should eat something. If she can't eat a normal diet, she should try to substitute the foods recommended for an insulin-dependent diabetic — ginger ale, soup, and the like. Liquids are particularly important to replace fluids lost in diarrhea. Since Jill has already taken her Orinase this morning, she must eat something today to prevent hypoglycemia. However, if she absolutely can't eat anything on subsequent days, she should stop taking her Orinase during those days.

Situation 5 — Pat

Tell Pat that consistently negative results are just as

dangerous as consistently high-positive results. They actually may predict future hypoglycemia. Optimally, urine test results should show a trace of glucose. To correct the consistently negative results, Pat should either decrease her insulin dose or increase her carbohydrate intake. The doctor can help her decide which course is best for her.

Situation 6 — Randy Thomas
Randy is experiencing symptoms of hyperglycemia in the afternoon, so his urine test results probably would be low before breakfast and lunch, very high before dinner, and somewhat reduced (though still high) before his bedtime snack. This pattern indicates either that Randy is eating way too much at lunch and in the afternoon, or that he isn't taking enough intermediate-acting insulin to see him through the afternoon and evening. In either case, he should be very concerned because this pattern could develop into ketoacidosis if uncorrected. Randy can correct the problem by sticking to his prescribed diet or by slightly increasing the dose of his Lente insulin, depending on his preference and his doctor's suggestion.

Situation 7 — Marvin Kissinger
Basically, Mr. Kissinger should simply stick to his usual diet and enjoy himself. Since German cooking often contains starchy vegetables, however, he should keep careful count of his carbohydrate intake. If he will be drinking ale or beer, he should eliminate 1½ bread exchanges for each 8-ounce glass. Dry wine is permissible with dinner, if taken in small quantities.

ANSWERS TO SKILLCHECK 3

Situation 1 — Frank Masullo
The doctor is checking for fatty accumulation beneath the skin, caused by repeated injections in the same site. Mr. Masullo may be using the same injection sites over and over because they've become fibrous and less sensitive. By using fibrous sites, though, Mr. Masullo isn't getting the full effect of his insulin, since fibrous areas absorb poorly.

Situation 2 — Edwin Allen
Based on Mr. Allen's confused, almost drunken behavior, you should suspect insulin-induced hypoglycemia. Mr. Allen may have compromised cerebral function due to his age and cerebral arteriosclerosis. Any slight decline in his blood sugar level would further impair his reasoning abilities, so that he might not recognize the early symptoms of hypoglycemia. The time of day may be another clue to Mr. Allen's condition. He would be most likely to experience hypoglycemia in the late afternoon, since his NPH

insulin would peak then. Mr. Allen may have skipped lunch and not have enough glucose to balance the insulin. Remember, too, that patients taking intermediate or long-acting insulin don't always show the classic symptoms of hypoglycemia. These insulins cause a slow decline in blood sugar, making cerebral symptoms more pronounced. Aphasia, uncoordinated movements, and psychotic behavior are common.

Situation 3 — Margaret Morris
Chances are Ms. Morris is in an ICU. Her condition is acute and demands constant attention, particularly attention to her blood-sugar level and her fluid intake and output. The first step in treatment would be to correct the insulin deficiency with I.V. insulin and to correct the dehydration, sodium depletion, and low blood volume with an I.V. of normal saline. After urinary output and renal blood flow were stabilized, she would receive I.V. potassium to correct the electrolyte imbalance and glucose to prevent her condition from going to the other extreme, hypoglycemia. But fluid output would have to be carefully monitored for adequate output before potassium could be added to the I.V. Because if output isn't adequate, the patient probably is retaining potassium; added potassium could cause dangerous cardiac arrhythmias.

Situation 4 — Andrew Sims
Don't be deceived by the fruity smell on Mr. Sims' breath. Although fruity breath and flushing may be consistent with DKA, four vital symptoms — strong pulse, profuse sweating, dilated pupils, and confusion and disorientation — point strongly to hypoglycemia. The fruity smell on Mr. Sims' breath could be alcohol or something else he had eaten. And the flushing may simply be Mr. Sims' individual way of responding to hypoglycemia. A blood-sugar test would probably be negative, confirming hypoglycemia.

Situation 5 — Jamie
The elevated blood sugar without accompanying acetones indicates HHNK. Jamie probably already had diabetes before he developed the throat infection. The infection increased his need for insulin, though, making his endogenous supply inadequate. Fever and vomiting contributed to Jamie's dehydration. Stress, insulin deficiency, and dehydration all combined to produce hyperglycemia. When superimposed on Jamie's preexisting diabetes, the hyperglycemia became exaggerated and turned into HHNK.

Situation 6 — Anne Loomis
Chances are her visual difficulties are only transitory. Anne is young and has just recently developed diabetes, so the possibility of permanent eye damage

from her diabetes, such as retinopathy, are remote. Many diabetics have trouble with their vision until their diabetes is stabilized because the accumulation of sorbital and fructose in the lens causes the eye to swell. When the glucose level returns to normal, the lens returns to its original shape and vision often improves.

Tell Anne that this process may take 6 to 8 weeks after she begins therapy. However, she should consult her doctor now to make sure she doesn't have any serious difficulty, such as a detached retina.

Situation 7 — George Franklin

Extensive dermatitis resembles burns in that the loss of skin integrity in both conditions results in an increased secretion of endogenous glucocorticoids. In Mr. Franklin's case, that natural process has been aggravated by high doses of exogenous steroids. The excess glucocorticoids have probably undercut his endogenous insulin's ability to metabolize glucose, resulting in hyperglycemia. If the glucocorticoids also suppressed release of ADH, osmotic diuresis probably led to dehydration. Mr. Franklin's I.V. fluids weren't enough to prevent dehydration. What's more, the fluids contain carbohydrates that would worsen his hyperglycemia. Although Mr. Franklin is receiving Lente insulin, it probably isn't enough to metabolize the glucose. Thus, the HHNK. To lower his blood sugar, give a supplement of Regular insulin.

Situation 8 — Vicki James

Actually, Vicki doesn't need her emergency kit. She could easily take 10 grams of carbohydrate — for instance, 3 ounces of Coca-Cola or 5 or 6 Life Savers — to correct her hypoglycemia. But if she must choose from her kit, she should select the dextrose wafer. (Glucagon, Glutose, and epinephrine all should be reserved for more advanced hypoglycemia.) Whether she uses a common carbohydrate or the dextrose wafer, though, she should follow it with a slower acting carbohydrate, such as peanut butter or bread. This combination will stem her immediate hypoglycemic reaction while providing ongoing glucose coverage.

ANSWERS TO SKILLCHECK 4

Situation 1 — Johnny Stover

Because he'll be getting more exercise than usual on his baseball days, Johnny will have to supplement his usual diet. Since he's a growing child, he should have more food at his noon meal and afternoon snack. He also should take a simple sugar to baseball practice, in case he misjudges the food-insulin balance and becomes hypoglycemic. Johnny also should delay his evening insulin injection until he's free from practice

and ready for supper. But he shouldn't decrease his insulin dose; otherwise, he might not have adequate control throughout the night. Although Johnny should be able to manage his diabetes with these adjustments, he also should make sure the coach or some other responsible adult with the team knows about his condition and can recognize all the signs of hypoglycemia. That person should keep Life Savers or a Coke on hand and know when to administer them.

Situation 2 — Mary Willis

Mrs. Willis has every right to be concerned about negative urine results. Since Mary is still developing neurologically, small amount of sugar in her urine (trace to 1+) would be better than hypoglycemia. Severe hypoglycemia, of course, could cause irreversible brain damage. Still, Mrs. Willis seems to be overly concerned about negative urine results. You should try to give her a more positive outlook on diabetes. Explain again the relationship of food and insulin to glucose levels and that proper therapy will keep Mary out of danger. If Mary refuses to eat exactly the foods on her meal plan, show her how to make substitutions from exchange lists. Also make sure she knows how to adjust food to coincide with activity levels. Finally, make sure she knows how to treat hypoglycemia with a high-glucose food or with glucagon. Mrs. Willis' anxiety will probably ease as she becomes more accustomed to the idea of Mary's diabetes and more proficient at caring for her. In the meantime, you could introduce her to well-adjusted mothers of other diabetic children; perhaps they could help her see Mary's diabetes as manageable.

Situation 3 — Terry

Try to get her to see her diabetes not as an illness but as a condition that simply needs to be controlled. Ask her to explain why she feels this way about her diabetes. If possible, arrange a group meeting with other diabetic teenagers or introduce Terry individually to other diabetic teenagers. If they have adjusted to their disease, they may change Terry's perspective; or, if they are having a similar reaction, simply talking it over may help both of them. You also might suggest consultation with a psych nurse, if one is available. The important step here is to get Terry to express her feelings. If she doesn't, she may stage a quiet rebellion by simply ignoring her diabetic therapy.

Situation 4 — Debby Rosen

From every indication, Debby can expect a normal, happy pregnancy, with little risk to herself or the baby. Debby qualifies as a Class C diabetic. She could develop hydramnios, toxemia, or urinary tract infections, as could any pregnant diabetic. But the chances are slight if she follows the doctor's orders and gets a check-up every two weeks; even if the conditions do develop, they can be treated. Since Debby is already managing her diabetes well with insulin, she won't have to change her therapy except to make minor adjustments in her insulin dose and diet to meet her changing needs throughout her pregnancy. The critical time of her pregnancy will occur after the 30th week; but the doctor will see her more often then and check her estriol level weekly to determine the best time for delivery. If all goes well, he'll probably induce her during the 36th or 37th week and she'll deliver naturally.

Situation 5 — Ed Phillips
Reassure Mr. Phillips that many blind diabetics live alone and do it quite well. Teach him how to measure his insulin injections and adminster them; you might suggest some injection devices, such as the copper sleeve, to help him guarantee accurate dose measurement. With some vision in his right eye, Mr. Phillips may be able to see when his insulin vials are empty. To be on the safe side, though, he should follow the practice of totally blind diabetics and use marbles to count doses. Mr. Phillips also may have enough vision to test his urine using color strips. If not, though, you should teach him the yeast method of testing urine. If Mr. Phillips won't be able to cook for himself, refer him to a local service agency, such as Meals on Wheels, an agency for the blind, or a local diabetes group. If none of these are available, you could help him arrange to dine with friends or at restaurants on a regular basis and to prepare simple meals at home.

Situation 6 — Eileen Shaunnessy
You could recommend any of several devices to help with self-injections. Many visually impaired diabetics prefer the Insulgage loading gauge because they can use it to vary dosages and to measure mixed doses. But if Ms. Shaunnessy must use a glass syringe for economic reasons, she might do better using the copper sleeve, which is designed specifically for a reusable syringe. If she uses U-40 or U-80 insulin and seldom varies the dose, she might prefer a Hill accurate dose syringe. Find out which devices best meet her specific needs. To remove air bubbles, Ms. Shaunnessy should draw up the insulin 3 times before injecting. If Ms. Shaunnessy still feels uneasy about giving herself injections, suggest that she have a nurse — friend, neighbor, or visiting nurse — check on her periodically.

Situation 7 — Nancy Byers
Advise Nancy to see her diabetologist right away. Stopping her oral hypoglycemic agent at this point might do more harm than good because, without it, her diabetes will be completely uncontrolled. That, of course, could be very harmful to the fetus. But the doctor will change Nancy to insulin for the duration of her pregnancy and during lactation.

Situation 8 — Ted Nichols
Ted can adjust to the trip quite easily if he makes these simple adjustments: Plan to eat extra food to cover his insulin dose during extra activity, or, if he can't tolerate the extra food, cut his insulin dose slightly. He should also carry a simple sugar with him in case he experiences hypoglycemic reactions. To be on the safe side, Ted should travel with someone who knows of his condition and can recognize and treat hypogylcemic reactions.

Situation 9 — Susan Hendricks
No. Clinitest results are unreliable during lactation because lactose spills into the urine, causing a false positive reading. Suggest that she get some Tes-Tape for urine testing; it tests specifically for glucose. If Tes-Tape results are positive, have her contact her doctor for further instructions.

ANSWERS TO SKILLCHECK 5

Situation 1 — Elliot Martin
Actually, Mr. Martin probably should increase his insulin dose. His anxiety coupled with the bodily insult of the surgery itself will have a diabetogenic effect. The sympathetic nervous system will release ACTH as well as the glucocorticoids of the adrenal cortex and epinephrine. Both ACTH and the glucocorticoids promote gluconeogenesis; epinephrine facilitates glycogenolysis. All of that results in an elevated blood sugar level, which requires more insulin. If Mr. Martin isn't eating, though, his blood sugar level may not rise much higher than his usual level. To determine exactly how much insulin he should take, you will have to check his urine every 4 to 6 hours.

Situation 2 — Francine Wilkes and Robert Upshaw
The five criteria are: severity of the diabetes, nature of the surgery, presence of diabetic complications, nondiabetic diagnosis, and the physician's preference in treatment.

Severity of the diabetes depends on the age of onset, stage of diabetes, and usual method of control. Nature of the surgery means whether it is minor or major, elective or emergency. The labels "minor" and "major" depend not only on the amount of physical trauma but also on the length of the procedure, anesthetic used, and the patient's psychological reaction to the surgery. (What normally is considered minor surgery may be considered major for some patients because they react so strongly to it, creating great stress and greatly altering glucose metabolism. Local or spinal anesthetics cause fewer metabolic disturbances than a general anesthetic.)

Diabetic complications include hypertension, peripheral vascular disease, foot decubiti, or a gangrenous toe. The nondiabetic diagnosis refers to co-existing conditions such as fistulae or cancer.

The physician's treatment preference refers to his chosen method of controlling the patient's diabetes, based on all the above information.

Situation 3 — Michael MacDonnald

Mr. MacDonnald sounds as though he's having a hypoglycemic reaction. He probably was told not to eat before leaving home this morning, but he may have taken his Tolinase to cover his food intake later. Because he has had to wait so long without food, his blood sugar has fallen below normal. You could confirm your suspicions with a quick blood sugar test. If his blood sugar is low, you should give him a quick source of glucose (Life Savers, Coca-Cola, etc.). He may have to reschedule his tests for another day. He could complete his test, however, if I.V. 50% glucose was given to increase his blood sugar.

Situation 4 — Saul Jaffe

Even though Mr. Jaffe normally would qualify as a mild diabetic, in his present serious condition he must be treated as a severe diabetic. He probably is receiving an I.V. of 5% dextrose in water and having his diabetes controlled with Regular insulin every 6 hours. You must check his urine to determine whether he needs a larger or smaller dose (5 additional units for each 1+ recorded). Mr. Jaffe probably has a Foley catheter. To obtain a specimen, do not disconnect the catheter. Instead, clamp the tubing for 15 to 30 minutes, allow-

ing the urine to collect in the bladder. Then clean the tubing with an alcohol wipe and aspirate a small amount of urine using a 25-gauge needle and syringe.

Before testing the specimen, check to see if Mr. Jaffe is receiving any other medications. Remember that large amounts of ascorbic acid, cephalosporins, Neg-gram, probenecid, other antibiotics, and salicylates will interfere with some urine tests. You may need to choose another urine test or test his blood sugar instead.

Situation 5 — Ron Kominsky

Since the surgery will be performed under a general anesthetic, you would keep Mr. Kominsky NPO the night before and the day of surgery. The doctor's orders would probably read as follows: One hour before the patient goes to the operating room, draw a STAT blood sugar. Then give ½ to ⅓ of his normal insulin dose subcutaneously and start an I.V. with 5% dextrose in water. If you are to administer a preop medication, such as morphine or demerol, give only ½ or ¾ the normal dose to avoid any nausea or vomiting. Nausea and vomiting could significantly lower his blood sugar, upsetting his diabetic control.

Situation 6 — Adele Wister

Despite the acetone in her urine, Ms. Wister sounds as though she's going into hypoglycemic coma (restlessness, diaphoresis). The ketones in her urine could stem from an infection, dehydration, or drugs she is given. A STAT blood sugar test will settle the question. But Ms. Wister also needs STAT treatment. Give her an injection of glucagon right after you draw the STAT blood. Remember that, when in doubt, you should give sugar to guard against the dire consequences of hypoglycemia.

APPENDICES

AMERICAN DIABETES ASSOCIATION EXCHANGE DIET

All foods appearing in italics are low-fat or non-fat.

Free Foods
There are certain foods you can use in unlimited amounts when planning your meals. Some of these include:

Diet calorie-free beverage	*Parsley*
Coffee	*Nutmeg*
Tea	*Lemon*
Bouillon without Fat	*Mustard*
Unsweetened Gelatin	*Chili Powder*
Unsweetened Pickles	*Onion Salt or Powder*
Salt and Pepper	*Horseradish*
Red Pepper	*Vinegar*
Paprika	*Mint*
Garlic	*Cinnamon*
Celery Salt	*Lime*

Forbidden Foods

sugar	jelly	chewing gum
candy	cookies	soft drinks
honey	syrup	pies
jam	condensed milk	cakes

List 1 Milk Exchanges
One exchange of milk contains 12 grams of carbohydrate, 8 grams of protein, a trace of fat and 80 calories.

This list shows the kinds and amounts of milk or milk products to use for one milk exchange. Low-fat and whole milk contain saturated fat.

Non-Fat Fortified Milk
  Skim or non-fat milk . . . . .1 cup
  Powdered (non-fat dry,
      before adding liquid) . . . . .⅓ cup
  Canned, evaporated – skim milk . . . . .½ cup
  Buttermilk made from skim milk . . . . .1 cup
  Yogurt made from skim milk
      (plain, unflavored) .1 cup
Low-Fat Fortified Milk
  1% fat fortified milk
      (omit ½ Fat Exchange) . . . . .1 cup
  2% fat fortified milk
      (omit 1 Fat Exchange) . . . . .1 cup
  Yogurt made from 2% fortified milk
      (plain, unflavored)
      (omit 1 Fat Exchange) . . . . .1 cup
Whole Milk (Omit 2 Fat Exchanges)
  Whole milk . . . . .1 cup
  Canned, evaporated whole milk . . . . .½ cup
  Buttermilk made from whole milk . . . . .1 cup
  Yogurt made from whole milk
      (plain, unflavored) .1 cup

List 2 Vegetable Exchanges

One exchange of vegetables contains about 5 grams of carbohydrate, 2 grams of protein and 25 calories. This list shows the kinds of vegetables to use for one vegetable exchange.

Asparagus ....½ cup
Bean Sprouts ....½ cup
Beets ....½ cup
Broccoli ....½ cup
Brussels Sprouts ....½ cup
Cabbage ....½ cup
Carrots ....½ cup
Cauliflower ....½ cup
Celery ....½ cup
Cucumbers ....½ cup
Eggplant ....½ cup
Green Pepper ....½ cup
Greens:
    Beet ....½ cup
    Chards ....½ cup
    Collards ....½ cup
    Dandelion ....½ cup
    Kale ....½ cup
    Mustard ....½ cup
    Spinach ....½ cup
    Turnip ....½ cup
Mushrooms ....½ cup
Okra ....½ cup
Onions ....½ cup
Rhubarb ....½ cup
Rutabaga ....½ cup
Sauerkraut ....½ cup
String Beans, green or yellow ......½ cup
Summer Squash ....½ cup
Tomatoes ....½ cup
Tomato Juice ....½ cup
Turnips ....½ cup
Vegetable Juice Cocktail ....½ cup
Zucchini ....½ cup

The following raw vegetables may be used as desired:

Chicory	Lettuce
Chinese Cabbage	Parsley
Endive	Radishes
Escarole	Watercress

(Starchy Vegetables are found in the Bread Exchange List)

List 3 Fruit Exchanges

One exchange of fruit contains 10 grams of carbohydrate and 40 calories. This list shows the kinds and amounts of fruits to use for one fruit exchange.

Apple ....1 small
Apple Juice ....⅓ cup
Applesauce (unsweetened) ....½ cup
Apricots, fresh ....2 medium
Apricots, dried ....4 halves

Banana ....½ small
Berries
    Blackberries ....½ cup
    Blueberries ....½ cup
    Raspberries ....½ cup
    Strawberries ....¾ cup
Cherries ....10 large
Cider ....⅓ cup
Dates 2
Figs, fresh 1
Figs, dried 1
Grapefruit ....½
Grapefruit Juice ....½ cup
Grapes 12
Grape Juice ....¼ cup
Mango ....½ small
Melon
    Cantaloupe ....½ small
    Honeydew ....⅛ medium
    Watermelon ....1 cup
Nectarine ....1 small
Orange ....1 small
Orange Juice ....¼ cup
Papaya ....¾ cup
Peach ....1 medium
Pear ....1 small
Persimmon, native ....1 medium
Pineapple ....½ cup
Pineapple Juice ....⅓ cup
Plums ....2 medium
Prunes ....2 medium
Prune Juice ....¼ cup
Raisins ....2 tbs.
Tangerine ....1 medium

Cranberries may be used as desired if no sugar is added.

List 4 Bread Exchanges

One exchange of bread contains 15 grams of carbohydrate, 2 grams of protein and 70 calories. This list shows the kinds and amounts of breads, cereals, starchy vegetables and prepared foods to use for one bread exchange.

Cereal
    Bran Flakes ....½ cup
    Other ready-to-eat
      unsweetened Cereal ....¾ cup
    Puffed Cereal (unfrosted) ....1 cup
    Cereal (cooked) ....½ cup
    Grits (cooked) ....½ cup
    Rice or Barley (cooked) ....½ cup
Pasta (cooked)
      Spaghetti, Noodles,
      Macaroni ....½ cup
Popcorn
    (popped, no fat added) ....3 cups

Cornmeal (dry) ....2 tbs.
Flour ....2½ tbs.
Wheat Germ ....¼ cup
Crackers
  Arrowroot 3
  Graham, 2½" sq. 2
  Matzoth, 4" x 6" ....½
  Oyster 20
  Pretzels, 3⅛" long x ⅛" dia. 25
  Rye Wafers, 2" x 3½" 3
  Saltines 6
  Soda, 2½" sq. 4
Dried Beans, Peas and Lentils
  Beans, Peas, Lentils
    (dried and cooked) ....½ cup
  Baked Beans, no pork
    (canned) ....¼ cup
Starchy Vegetables
  Corn ....⅓ cup
  Corn on Cob ....1 small
  Lima Beans ....½ cup
  Parsnips ....⅔ cup
  Peas, Green (canned or frozen) ....½ cup
  Potato, White ....1 small
  Potato (mashed) ....½ cup
  Pumpkin ....¾ cup
  Winter Squash,
    Acorn or Butternut ....½ cup
  Yam or Sweet Potato ....¼ cup
Prepared Foods
  Biscuit 2" dia.
    (omit 1 Fat Exchange) 1
  Corn Bread, 2" x 2" x 1"
    (omit 1 Fat Exchange) 1
  Corn Muffin, 2" dia.
    (omit 1 Fat Exchange) 1
  Crackers, round butter type
    (omit 1 Fat Exchange) 5
  Muffin, plain small
    (omit 1 Fat Exchange) 1
  Potatoes, French Fried,
    Length 2" to 3½"
    (omit 1 Fat Exchange) 8
  Potato or Corn Chips
    (omit 2 Fat Exchanges) 15
  Pancake, 5" x ½"
    (omit 1 Fat Exchange) 1
  Waffle, 5" x ½"
    (omit 1 Fat Exchange) 1

List 5 Meat Exchanges

(Lean Meat)
One exchange of lean meat (1 oz.) contains 7 grams of protein, 3 grams of fat and 55 calories. This list shows the kinds and amounts of lean meat and other protein-rich foods to use for one low-fat meat exchange.

Beef:
  Baby beef (very lean), chipped beef,
  chuck, flank steak, tenderloin, plate ribs,
  plate skirt steak, round (bottom, top),
  all cuts rump, spare ribs, tripe ....1 oz.
Lamb:
  Leg, rib, sirloin, loin (roast and chops),
  shank, shoulder ....1 oz.
Pork:
  Leg (whole rump, center shank)
  ham, smoked (center slices) ....1 oz.
Veal:
  Leg, loin, rib, shank, shoulder,
  cutlets ....1 oz.
Poultry:
  Meat without skin of chicken, turkey,
  cornish hen, guinea hen,
  pheasant ....1 oz.
Fish:
  Any fresh or frozen ....1 oz.
  canned salmon, tuna, mackerel, crab
  and lobster ....¼ cup
  clams, oysters, scallops,
  shrimp ....5 or 1 oz.
  sardines, drained 3
Cheeses containing less than 5%
  butterfat ....1 oz.
Cottage cheese, dry and 2%
  butterfat ....¼ cup
Dried beans and peas (omit 1
  bread exchange) ....½ cup

List 5 Meat Exchanges

(Medium-Fat Meat)
For each exchange of medium-fat meat omit ½ fat exchange. This list shows the kinds and amounts of medium-fat meat and other protein-rich foods to use for one medium-fat meat exchange.

Beef:
  Ground (15% fat), corned beef (canned),
  rib eye, round (ground commercial) ....1 oz.
Pork:
  Loin (all cuts tenderloin),
  shoulder arm (picnic),
  shoulder blade, Boston butt,
  Canadian bacon, boiled ham ....1 oz.
Liver, heart, kidney and sweetbreads
  (these are high in cholesterol) ....1 oz.
Cottage cheese, creamed ....¼ cup
Cheese:
  Mozzarella, ricotta, farmer's cheese,
    neufchatel ....1 oz.
  Parmesan ....3 tbs.
Egg (high in cholesterol) 1
Peanut butter (omit 2 additional
  fat exchanges) ....2 tbs.

List 5 Meat Exchanges
(High-Fat Meat)

For each exchange of high-fat meat omit 1 fat exchange. This list shows the kinds and amounts of high-fat meat and other protein-rich foods to use for one high-fat meat exchange.

Beef:
Brisket, corned beef (brisket), ground beef (more than 20% fat), hamburger (commercial), chuck (ground commercial), roasts (rib), steaks (club and rib) ....1 oz.

Lamb:
Breast ....1 oz.

Pork:
Spare ribs, loin (back ribs), pork (ground), country style ham, deviled ham ....1 oz.

Veal:
Breast ....1 oz.

Poultry:
Capon, duck (domestic), goose ....1 oz.

Cheese:
Cheddar types ....1 oz.

Cold cuts ....4½" x ⅛" slice

Frankfurter ....1 small

List 6 Fat Exchanges

One exchange of fat contains 5 grams of fat and 45 calories. This list shows the kinds and amounts of fat-containing foods to use for one fat exchange.

*Margarine, soft, tub or stick** ....1 tsp.
*Avocado (4" in diameter)*** ....⅛

Oil
Corn, Cottonseed, Safflower,
Soy, Sunflower ....1 tsp.

*Oil, Olive** ....1 tsp.
*Oil, Peanut** ....1 tsp.
*Olives** ....5 small
*Almonds** ....10 whole
*Pecans** ....2 large
*Peanuts**
Spanish ....20 whole
Virginia ....10 whole
Walnuts ....6 small
*Nuts, other** ....6 small

Margarine, regular stick ....1 tsp.
Butter ....1 tsp.
Bacon fat ....1 tsp.
Bacon, crisp ....1 strip
Cream, light ....2 tbs.
Cream, sour ....2 tbs.
Cream, heavy ....1 tbs.
Cream Cheese ....1 tbs.
French dressing*** ....1 tbs.
Italian dressing*** ....1 tbs.
Lard ....1 tsp.
Mayonnaise*** ....1 tsp.
Salad dressing, mayonnaise type*** ....2 tsp.
Salt pork ....¾" cube

*Made with corn, cottonseed, safflower, soy or sunflower oil only
**Fat content is primarily monounsaturated
***If made with corn, cottonseed, safflower, soy or sunflower oil, can be used on fat modified diet

DRUG INTERACTIONS WITH ORAL HYPOGLYCEMIC AGENTS

Interacting Drug	Oral Agents	Effect
A		
acetazolamide (Diamox)	sulfonylureas only	hyperglycemia
alcohol	all	hypoglycemia (acute ingestion only); hyperglycemia (chronic ingestion only); Antabuse-like reaction with sulfonylureas only; lactic acidosis with phenformin only
allopurinol (Zyloprim)	sulfonylureas only	hypoglycemia
anabolic steroid hormones (Adroyd, Anavar*, Dianabol*, Winstrol, etc.)	all	hypoglycemia
aspirin	all	hypoglycemia
B		
barbiturates (Amytal, Nembutal, phenobarbital, Seconal, Tuinal, etc.)	sulfonylureas only	prolonged sedation
C		
chloramphenicol (Chloromycetin)	sulfonylureas, except acetohexamide	hypoglycemia
clofibrate (Atromid-S)	sulfonylureas only	hypoglycemia
corticosteroids (Celestone, cortisone, Decadron, hydrocortisone, Kenalog, Medrol, prednisolone, prednisone, Valisone, etc.)	all	hyperglycemia; impairs glucose tolerance
coumarin anticoagulants (Coumadin, Dicumarol)	sulfonylureas only	hypoglycemia; increased anti-coagulant effect for several days followed by decreased anticoagulant effect
cyclophosphamide (Cytoxan)	sulfonylureas only	hypoglycemia
D		
dextrothyroxine (Choloxin)	all	hyperglycemia
diazoxide (Hyperstat)	all	hyperglycemia; hypokalemia (replacement of potassium may return blood sugar to normal)
E		
epinephrine (Adrenalin, SusPhrine)	all	hyperglycemia

estrogens (Menest*, Ogen, Premarin, ORAL CONTRACEPTIVES)	all	hyperglycemia; hypokalemia (replacement of potassium may return blood sugar to normal)
ethacrynic acid (Edecrin)	all	hyperglycemia; hypokalemia (replacement of potassium may return blood sugar to normal)

F

furosemide (Lasix)	all	hyperglycemia

G

glucagon	all	hyperglycemia
guanethidine (Ismelin)	all	hypoglycemia

I

indomethacin (Indocin)	sulfonylureas only	hyperglycemia
insulin	all	hypoglycemia
isoniazid (INH)	sulfonylureas only	hyperglycemia with large doses only

L

levothyroxine (Synthroid)	all	hyperglycemia

M

marijuana	all	hyperglycemia
methyldopa (Aldomet)	sulfonylureas only	serious blood dyscrasias
methysergide (Sansert)		hypoglycemia
monoamine oxidase inhibitors (Eutonyl, Marplan, Nardil, Parnate)	all except acetohexamide	hypoglycemia; may release false adrenergic neurotransmitter

N

nicotinic acid (Niacin)	sulfonylureas only	hyperglycemia with large doses only

O

oxyphenbutazone (Tandearil, Oxalid*)	sulfonylureas only	hypoglycemia

P

phenformin (DBI, Metrol)	all	hypoglycemia
phenothiazines (Compazine, Mellaril, Phenergan, Prolixin*, Sparine, Stelazine, Temaril*, Thorazine, etc.)	all	hyperglycemia
phenylbutazone (Butazolidin, Azolid)	sulfonylureas only	hypoglycemia
phenytoin (Dilantin)	all	hyperglycemia

probenecid (Benemid)	sulfonylureas only	hypoglycemia
propranolol (Inderal)	all	hypoglycemia

R

rifampin (Rifadin, Rimactane)	sulfonylureas except acetohexamide	hyperglycemia

S

salicylates	all	hypoglycemia
sulfonamides (Gantrisin, Gantanol, Bactrim, Septra, Thiosulfil)	sulfonylureas only	hypoglycemia; increased blood levels of sulfonamide (may be beneficial)
sulfonylureas (Diabinese, Dymelor, Orinase, Tolinase*)	all	hypoglycemia

T

tetracyclines (Achromycin, Aureomycin, Declomycin, Minocin, Sumycin, Terramycin, Vibramycin)	sulfonylureas only	hypoglycemia
thiazide diuretics (Diuril, Esidrix, HydroDIURIL, Oretic*, Renese, etc.)	all	hyperglycemia; hypokalemia (replacement of potassium may return blood sugar to normal)
thyroid hormone	all	hyperglycemia; increased thyroid effect
triamterene (Dyrenium)	all	hyperglycemia; hypokalemia (replacement of potassium may return blood sugar to normal)

Not available in Canada

INDEX

HHNK. See *Hyperglycemic hyperosmolar nonketotic coma.*
Hill Accurate Dosage Syringe, 178, 179
Hormone(s), 161, 172
Hospitalization, of child, 160, 166
Hydramnios, 169, 170
Hydration, rate, 148
  solution, 148
Hydroxybutyrate urine tests, 81-82
Hyperalimentation therapy
  HHNK from, 144, 146
  postoperative, 197
Hyperbilirubinemia, 168
Hyperglycemia
  in ketoacidosis, 132
  in oral therapy, 44
  in pregnancy, 169
  postoperative, 197
  rebound, 120
  symptoms, 16, 44, 140
Hyperglycemic hyperosmolar nonketotic coma (HHNK), 141-153
  blood urea nitrogen levels in, 150
  central nervous system manifestation, 151
  coma, in, 150
  dehydration in, 147-150
  hydration maintenance in, 151
  hypokalemia in, 149
  insulin levels and, 151
  ketoacidosis versus, 134, 151, 153
  ketone bodies, 151
  mortality rate, 141, 145, 151
  nonketosis in, 150
  nursing care, 151-152
  onset, 145
  physiologic aspects, 144
  postoperative, 198
  precipitating factors, 144, 146
  prevention, 151-153
  signs and symptoms, 128, 143, 143t, 145
  serum growth hormone and cortical levels, 151
  sodium deficit in, 147
  treatment, 142, 147
  water intoxication in, 153
Hyperinsulinism prevention, 52
Hyperkalemia, EKG of, 136
Hyperosmolality, 146

in HHNK, 147-150
  treatment, 147, 149
Hyperstat, 23
Hyperthyroidism, 22
Hypnotic drugs, 45
Hypocalcemia, in babies, 168
Hypoglycemia. See also *Insulin reaction.*
  brain damage from, 117, 195
  drug-induced, 119
  drug-potentiated, 42
  from hypoglycemic agents, 42
  in children, 163, 168
  in kidney failure, 108
  in surgery, 190
  patient ignorance of, 116-117
  postoperative, 195
  precipitating factors, 42
  signs and symptoms, 17, 43, 117, 118, 121, 122
  treatment, 119, 125
Hypoglycemic agents, 35-48
  alcohol intolerance from, 45
  allergies to, 37
  barriers to, 37
  cardiac death and, 36
  comparison of, 39t
  contraindications, 35-37, 41
  convenience, 35
  diet with, 36, 40
  discovery of, 44
  dosages, 41
  drug incompatibilities, 45
  during breast-feeding, 174
  effectiveness, 47
  exercise and, 36, 40
  fasting and, 41
  fever and, 37
  foot care and, 41
  for children, 160
  foreign equivalents of, 39, 92
  hypoglycemia from, 44
  in elderly, 37
  insulin versus, 35
  lactic acidosis from, 37, 44
  physiologic action, 37, 118
  pregnancy and, 37, 172
  risks, 42-46
  selection of, 39
  urine testing with, 41
Hypokalemia, 136, 149
Hypovolemia, 146

I

Identification tags, 62, 89, 166
Illness(es), nondiabetic

carbohydrates and, 84
diet in, 85
effects on diabetics, 83-88
liquid intake in, 84
preparations for, 85, 86
short-term versus long-term, 86-88
Immunization, before trip, 89
Impotence, 111
Incontinence, 109, 110
Infection(s), 16, 195, 201
  blood sugar and, 146
  foot, 114
  hypoglycemic agents and, 37
  of soft tissue, 189
  pain as warning of, 195
  postoperative, 196
  skin, 102
  urinary, 108, 109
Injection sites, 65-66
  reactions at, 55, 104
  vascularity of, 51
Instant Glucose, 126
Insulgage Loading Gauge, 178, 179
Insulin, 49-52
  action of, 46, 50, 50t
  administration, 51, 52
    during surgery, 191, 193
  antagonists, in children, 161
  blood sugar response to, 14, 53, 54
  Canadian, 50
  concentrations of, 50, 51, 64
  daily use of, 49-55
  discovery of, 191
  dosage(s)
    during jet flight, 93
    errors in, 123
    food intake and, 200
    in alcoholism, 119
    in children, 160, 163, 164
    increase of, 120
    in kidney failure, 119
    in liver disease, 119
    modification, 54
    renal glucose threshold and, 24
  drawing up, 67-68
  examination of color, 52
  for protein allergy, 50
  inefficient use of, 17
  injection(s), 52, 69
    in blind, 176-180
    in children, 162-163
    sites for, 65-66

ABOUT THE AUTHORS

Gail B. Askew, PharmD, is an inpatient staff pharmacist at the University of California at Ervine. Dr. Askew received her PharmD from the University of Southern California School of Pharmacy. She is a member of the American Society of Hospital Pharmacists.

Barbara Christman, RN, MSN, assistant professor of medical-surgical nursing at Vanderbilt University in Tennessee, is president of the American Association of Diabetes Educators. She also works as clinical specialist in diabetes at Vanderbilt's Medical Center.

Veronica Engle, RN, is a former diabetes nurse practitioner at Veterans Administration Hospital in Madison, Wisconsin. Ms. Engle holds a BSN from the University of Wisconsin-Madison where presently she is a graduate student.

Catherine Garofano, RN, BS, works as clinical nurse in the Endocrine-Metabolic Unit in Hahnemann Medical College, Philadelphia. For eleven years she was associated with the Peter Bent Brigham Hospital in Boston where she was head nurse of the Female Medical Ward Pavilion.

Diana W. Guthrie, RN, MSPH, is a diabetes nurse specialist and assistant professor at Wichita State University in Kansas. Mrs. Guthrie has BSN and MSN degrees from the University of Missouri and is a fellow in the American Academy of Nursing.

Richard A. Guthrie, MD, is professor and chairman of the Department of Pediatrics at the Wichita State University branch of the Kansas University Medical School. As an endocrinologist specializing in diabetes in children, Dr. Guthrie is on the Board of Directors of the American Diabetes Association.

Susan Kaufmann, RN, BS, is a coordinator of teaching nurses at Joslin Diabetes Foundation in Boston. Mrs. Kaufmann is a member of the American Diabetes Association's committee on food and nutrition. She is presently enrolled in the Health Education master's program at Boston University.

Kenneth I. Letcher, PharmD, is director of Pharmaceutical Services at Presbyterian Hospital of Pacific Medical Center and St. Luke's in San Francisco. He earned his PharmD from the University of California School of Pharmacy.

Edwina A. McConnell, RN, MS, has a BS degree from Boston University and earned her MS from the University of Colorado. Ms. McConnell is the assistant director of surgical nursing at Madison General Hospital in Madison, Wisconsin, and has served as an ICU staff nurse and head nurse on a surgical floor.

Rita Nemchik, RN, MS, a former coordinator of Patient and Community Health Education at St. Francis Hospital in Trenton, now serves as assistant director of education at Pennsylvania Hospital located in Philadelphia.

Michael L. O'Connor, MD, is associate professor of pathology and director of clinical laboratories at Wake Forest University's Bowman Gray School of Medicine. Dr. O'Connor's articles have appeared in the AMERICAN JOURNAL OF CLINICAL PATHOLOGY AND CLINICAL BIOCHEMISTRY.

Judith C. Petrokas, RN, serves as diabetic clinical nurse specializing in education at the Miami Valley Hospital in Dayton, Ohio, where formerly she coordinated a continuing care unit. She is a member of the Board of Trustees of the Dayton Diabetic Association.

Joyce Schulz, RN, is a diploma graduate of Montreal General Hospital. She is nurse consultant for the Minneapolis Society for the Blind and has contributed to the pamphlet BLINDNESS AND DIABETES, published by the American Foundation for the Blind.

Delores Schumann, RN, MS, earned a diploma from Miami Valley Hospital School of Nursing in Dayton Ohio, a BS from Ohio State University, and an MS from Boston University. She is a lecturer in the School of Nursing, Graduate Nursing Division at the University of Wisconsin-Madison.

Marie Williams, BA, MSW, is a supervisor of social science for the Minneapolis Society for the Blind. Mrs. Williams received her degree from the University of Minnesota. She is a member of the American Association of Workers for the Blind and has contributed to THE NEW OUTLOOK FOR THE BLIND magazine.

Karen Witt, RN, a former clinical nurse specialist in respiratory care at the University of Wisconsin, has also worked as a staff nurse, head nurse, and public health nurse. Mrs. Witt is a member of the Wisconsin Respiratory Care Society and author of the Wisconsin Dial-Access tape, TRACHEOSTOMY CARE.

Lawrence W. Wolfe, BSc, RPh, is adjunct clinical instructor at the Temple University School of Pharmacy and clinical pharmacist at Temple University Hospital in Philadelphia. His special area of interest is metabolic diseases, especially hyperalimentation and diabetes.